Best Practices in Child and Adolescent Behavioral Health Care

Series Editor

Fred R. Volkmar
Yale University
New Haven, CT, USA

Best Practices in Child and Adolescent Behavioral Health Care series explores a range of topics relevant to primary care providers in managing a broad range of child and adolescent mental health problems. These include specific disorders, such as anxiety; relevant topics in related disciplines, including psychological assessment, communication assessment, and disorders; and such general topics as management of psychiatric emergencies. The series aims to provide primary care providers with leading-edge information that enables best-care management of behavioral health issues in children and adolescents. The volumes published in this series provide concise summaries of the current research base (i.e., what is known), best approaches to diagnosis and assessment, and leading evidence-based management and treatment strategies. The series also provides information and analysis that primary care providers need to understand how to interpret and implement best treatment practices and enable them to interpret and implement recommendations from specialists for children and effectively monitor interventions.

More information about this series at http://www.springer.com/series/15955

Patricia A. Prelock • Tiffany L. Hutchins

Clinical Guide to Assessment and Treatment of Communication Disorders

Springer

Patricia A. Prelock
College of Nursing & Health Sciences
University of Vermont
Burlington, VT, USA

Tiffany L. Hutchins
Department of Communication
Sciences & Disorders
University of Vermont
Burlington, VT, USA

ISSN 2523-7128 ISSN 2523-7136 (electronic)
Best Practices in Child and Adolescent Behavioral Health Care
ISBN 978-3-030-06611-6 ISBN 978-3-319-93203-3 (eBook)
https://doi.org/10.1007/978-3-319-93203-3

Softcover re-print of the Hardcover 1st edition 2018

This Springer imprint is published by the registered company Springer Nature Switzerland AG
The registered company address is: Gewerbestrasse 11, 6330 Cham, Switzerland

We would like to dedicate this book to our families for their unending support of our work.

Series Editor Preface

Primary care providers are increasingly asked to assume a great role in both the diagnosis and continued management and care of children with a range of developmental and behavioral problems. This is an increased role, both in early diagnosis and treatment, which involves coordination with evaluators and care providers from a range of disciplines. Challenges arise on all sides and range from learning to understand each other's specialized terminology to practical issues of access to quality evaluations and treatment. The myriad of complexities in dealing with insurance plans only adds to the burden of parents and care providers. Services vary considerably from place to place. Fortunately, mandates for services in most countries mean that schools provide important rehabilitative services. However, even here, there is an important role for the primary care providers in the coordination of care. For mental health and developmental problems, the tripartite system of care (self-pay, state-supported insurance, and private service) poses other obstacles for obtaining specialized medical assessments and, in particular, mental health services. The use of the medical home model (Sheldrick & Perrin, 2010) provides an important overarching plan for these efforts but still requires a basic understanding of these conditions on the part of primary care practitioners.

In this series, our goal is to provide primary care physicians, nurse practitioners, and other related professionals in the field with practical, evidence-based guides for a range of topics concerned with developmental and mental health disorders. In this first volume of the series, Drs. Patricia Prelock and Tiffany Hutchins provide a clinical guide to understanding and treating communication disorders in conditions like autism, where social communication problems are so much a focus of treatment.

Problems in communication include a range of conditions – from problems in articulation to broader problems in expressive and receptive language, and in the complex world of social language use. Early detection and intervention are often the key to successful treatment. Even though questions about speech delays and language problems are very commonly mentioned by parents, many medical care providers have little understanding of these conditions as well as the work of speech-language pathologists in their assessment and treatment. While excellent specialized textbooks on the topic are available (e.g., Paul, Norbury, & Gosse, 2018), straightforward practical guides have not been so readily available.

In this volume, Prelock and Hutchins give readers a basic understanding of the typical pattern of communication development in children and adolescents. This volume describes screening and assessment protocols and when referrals should be made for such assessments. It also helps practitioners on how to talk about intervention and educational practices with other caregivers and parents. This volume, the first in the series, sets a high standard which we hope to maintain in subsequent volumes.

Fred R. Volkmar

Irving B. Harris Professor of Child Psychiatry,
Pediatrics, and Psychology,
Yale University School of Medicine
New Haven, CT, USA

References

Paul, R., Norbury, C., & Gosse, C. (2018). *Language disorders from infancy through adolescence: listening, speaking, reading, writing, and communicating*. St. Louis, MO: Elsevier.

Sheldrick, R. C., & Perrin, E. C. (2010). Medical home services for children with behavioral health conditions. *Journal of Developmental & Behavioral Pediatrics*, 31(2), 92–99.

Acknowledgments

We would like to acknowledge the children with communication disorders and their families who have taught us an incredible amount about the challenges they face in sharing their messages and understanding the messages of others. A special thank you to Dr. Shelley Velleman for her contribution to the chapter on "Children with Speech Disorders" and to Dr. Elizabeth Adams for her guidance and feedback as an audiologist on the "Children with Hearing Loss" chapter.

Contents

About the Authors

Patricia A. Prelock Ph.D., CCC-SLP, BRS-CL, is Professor and Dean in the College of Nursing and Health Sciences and Professor of Pediatrics in the College of Medicine at the University of Vermont. Dr. Prelock coordinates parent training programs designed for caregivers of children with ASD and has been awarded more than 11 million dollars in university, state, and federal funding as a PI or Co-PI to develop innovations in interdisciplinary training supporting children and youth with neurodevelopmental disabilities and their families, to facilitate training in speech-language pathology, and to support her intervention work in ASD. She has over 180 publications and 528 peer-reviewed and invited presentations/keynotes in the areas of autism and other neurodevelopmental disabilities, collaboration, IPE, leadership, and language learning disabilities. Dr. Prelock received the University of Vermont's Kroepsch-Maurice Excellence in Teaching Award in 2000 and was named an ASHA Fellow in 2000 and a University of Vermont Scholar in 2003. In 2011, she was named the Cecil and Ida Green Honors Professor Visiting Scholar at Texas Christian University and in 2015 was named a Distinguished Alumna of the University of Pittsburgh. In 2016, she received the ASHA Honors of the Association, and in 2017 she was named a Distinguished Alumna of Cardinal Mooney High School. Dr. Prelock is a Board Certified Specialist in Child Language and was named a Fellow in the National Academies of Practice (NAP) in speech-language pathology in 2018. She was the 2013 President for the American Speech-Language Hearing Association and is leading the development of the University of Vermont Integrative Health Program.

Tiffany Hutchins Ph.D., is Associate Professor at the University of Vermont. Her research has centered on the relationships from mother-child interaction strategies to social cognition and child cognitive and language development. She has developed and validated new measures of theory of mind (see https://www.theoryofmindinventory.com/) that can be used in research and practice with typically developing individuals and those with developmental disabilities. She is currently investigating the efficacy of story-based interventions to remediate the core deficits of autism spectrum disorder (ASD). With the use of eye-tracking technology, she has established a new program of research to examine how individuals with ASD allocate visual attention when viewing face stimuli. Dr. Hutchins also examines social cognition or theory of mind in oral and late-signing children with hearing loss. She teaches courses in the development of spoken language, cognition and language, measurement in communication sciences, and language disorders.

Chapter 1
Overview of Communication Disorders

Introduction

In this chapter we provide a brief introduction to what a communication disorder is, an explanation of the various terms used to describe communication disorders, and a description of the types of communication disorders primary care providers are most likely to see. This chapter will also outline the content focus for each of the chapters that follow. Although communication disorders exist across the life span, the focus of this chapter and book is on the communication disorders most often seen in children and youth.

What Is a Communication Disorder?

The ability to communicate is critical as it is the primary means of sharing our thoughts, ideas, and feelings across the life span. A communication disorder disrupts an individual's ability to exchange meaning with another when sending and/or receiving information. It can be congenital, meaning an individual is born with a disorder that impacts communication (e.g., cerebral palsy, deafness), or it can be acquired, meaning something happened after birth that affected communication (e.g., traumatic brain injury, meningitis) (Gillam & Marquardt, 2016). Communication disorders are also described as organic, suggesting a physical cause, or functional, suggesting an unknown cause.

Nearly 46 million people have a communication disorder that impacts their ability to talk and/or hear (National Institute on Deafness and Other Communication Disorders, 2015b). A national survey of children with communication disorders indicates that nearly 1 in 12 children are diagnosed with a communication disorder (7.7%) between the ages of 3 and 17 affecting speech, voice, language, and/or

P. A. Prelock, T. L. Hutchins, *Clinical Guide to Assessment and Treatment of Communication Disorders*, Best Practices in Child and Adolescent Behavioral Health Care, https://doi.org/10.1007/978-3-319-93203-3_1

Table 1.1 US prevalence of communication disorders in children aged 3–17[a]

Type of disorder	Percent of occurrence (%)
Speech	5.5
Language	3.3
Voice	1.4
Swallowing	0.9

[a]Black, Vahratian, & Hoffman (2015). Communication Disorders and Use of Intervention Services among Children Aged 3–17: United States, 2012

Table 1.2 US demographic characteristics of children with communication disorders[a]

Demographics	Percent
Boys	9.6
Girls	5.7
3–6-year-olds	11
7–10-year-olds	9.3
11–17-year-olds	4.9
Black	9.6
White	7.8
Hispanic	6.9

[a]Communication Disorders and Use of Intervention Services among Children Aged 3–17: United States, 2012

swallowing with about 50% of these children receiving intervention (*The Asha Leader*, 2015a, b). Table 1.1 highlights the occurrence of particular communication disorders in children.

Notably, more than one third of the youngest children (ages 3–10) and approximately a quarter of older children (ages 11–17) have more than one of the disorders noted above. Table 1.2 displays the demographic characteristics of children with communication disorders, revealing that boys and black children are more likely to have a greater occurrence of communication problems.

Of the almost 8% of children with communication disorders, those with speech (67.6%) or language problems (66.8%) occur more often than those with voice (22.8%) or swallowing (12.7%) disorders. Knowing that children with language disorders have poorer academic achievement than those with articulation disorders alone (Hall & Tomblin, 1978) and are more likely to have poor academic outcomes including reading disabilities (Aram & Nation, 1980), it is critical to refer identified children to a speech-language pathologist who can facilitate an appropriate assessment and make a plan for intervention in collaboration with the family and primary care provider.

There also appears to be a cultural influence in the access to services for children with communication disorders with white children (60.1%) receiving intervention services at a greater rate than Hispanic (47.3%) or black (45.85%) children. Further, differences in access to intervention services also exist for boys (59.4%) vs. girls (47.8%) with communication disorders (*The Asha Leader*, 2015a, b). It is important, therefore, that primary care providers remain vigilant in their screening of potential communication disorders in the patients or clients they see and their referral to a speech-language pathologist.

What Terms Are Used to Describe a Communication Disorder?

Primary care providers may hear any number of terms to describe a child with a communication disorder. The World Health Organization (2011) uses the word "impairment" to refer to those who have experienced a loss of function or an abnormality in structure. As an example, a person with a hearing loss may have difficulty hearing but that does not automatically equate to someone who is unable to function well in society. Generally, a discussion of impairment suggests we want to understand a person's strengths and challenges and what we can do to address these. In contrast, a "disorder" often refers to a loss of competence in addressing daily needs. If we keep with the example of a person with a hearing loss, the individual's hearing may hinder that individual from being able to talk on the telephone even when aided. Typically, a discussion of *disability* indicates that we want to understand to what extent an individual can access daily activities when provided with some level of support.

The term *communication disorder* has been used synonymously with impairment and disability but is most often used to indicate some diminished communication structure or function (Gillam & Marquardt, 2016). There are also times when a communication disorder may be seen as a "disability or handicap" in that it interferes with an individual's ability to actively participate in his/her environment.

Primary care providers also may see patients or clients with a *communication difference*, that is, a communication ability that is different from what it typically encountered. For example, a child whose native language is French and who learned English as a second language is not necessarily expected to have the same ease learning English as she did with French. A child who is learning English as a second language may require some extra time and help in learning English, particularly in social and educational contexts. Unless there is a communication impairment characterized by the loss of function or structure, children's limited proficiency in an emerging second language should not be identified as a communication disorder, and they should not be referred to a speech-language pathologist.

What Types of Communication Disorders Are Likely to Be Seen in a Primary Care or Pediatric Practice?

Typically, communication disorders are described as speech disorders, language disorders, or hearing disorders. Speech disorders are the result of an interruption in speech production and usually fall in one of three categories: articulation and phonological disorders, fluency disorders, and voice disorders (Gillam & Marquardt, 2016). For preschoolers the prevalence for speech disorders is 8–9%, with 5% of this population demonstrating noticeable speech disorders when they reach first grade (National Institute on Deafness and Other Communication Disorders, 2015b). Language disorders are the result of a disruption in the comprehension and/or expression of meaning through words and sentences. Language disorders occur in three primary categories: developmental language disorders that occur during childhood, acquired language disorders that can occur during childhood and adulthood, and dementia which usually occurs in older adults. Between 6 and 8 million people are reported to have a language disorder in the USA (National Institute on Deafness and Other Communication Disorders, 2015a).

A child's early experiences and connections to caregivers are critical for developing communication (Center on the Developing Child at Harvard University, 2012). Some children living in poverty may be at risk for lower language because of their lack of access to a stimulating language environment in infancy and the toddler years (Hart & Risley, 1995). In fact, there is a gap in the expressive language development of children from poor socioeconomic backgrounds versus those from higher socioeconomic backgrounds, and this gap can be identified as early as 18 months (Fernald, Marchman, & Weisleder, 2013). By 3 years of age, this gap is even larger with children from upper socioeconomic status (SES) having an expressive vocabulary three times larger than children coming from homes with lower income (Hart & Risley, 1995). Once they reach kindergarten, children from lower SES may already be disadvantaged in both their achievement and the lack of school quality they are likely to experience (Lee & Burkam, 2002). These results persist in elementary school for both language development and academic achievement (Walker, Greenwood, Hart & Carta, 1994).

It is important that primary care providers understand the context in which young children are experiencing and learning language so that appropriate referrals to language-rich daycare and preschool environments are made. It is also important to guide families in the kinds of rich language interactions that will most likely facilitate their children's communication development and play. For example, toy selection might be one consideration in a well-child visit to support the social interaction, play, and language development of young children at risk. In fact, Porter (2012) reported on the impact of toys children are exposed to in play, explaining that toys with specific uses like wind-up toys and coloring books provide less opportunity for creativity and are less likely to support sociodramatic play – an important environment for language development. In contrast, toys that are more open-ended and can lead to multiple uses such as blocks and play-doh are likely to facilitate play, interaction, and language development.

Overview of the Book Chapters

In Chap. 2, *An Introduction to Typical Communication Development*, the reader is given an overview of the development of language to provide a basic understanding of typical development. More specifically, the universal speech and language milestones that are known to emerge in late infancy and toddlerhood are described and some discussion about how these early developments are shaped in early and later childhood are also discussed. Chapter 3, *Approaches to Screening and Diagnosis*, outlines the principles for screening and diagnosis for the most common communication disorders in children and highlights popular screening and assessment tools for speech and language functioning.

Chapter 4, *Principles Guiding Intervention and Educational Practices*, focuses on a discussion of family-centered care in the context of the medical home and integrated models of service delivery which are culturally competent and developmentally appropriate. Care plan development is briefly reviewed as it relates to the development of individual family service plans (IFSPs) and individual educational plans (IEPs). This chapter also includes a discussion of needed collaborations among related service providers and how to prioritize and streamline care coordination across agencies and educational programs.

In Chap. 5, *Understanding Late Talkers*, consideration is given to determining when to "wait and watch" and how to identify risk factors for disordered development in those children with a communication delay as well as knowing when to refer and how to talk with families about their child's communication development. Children with communication delays may resolve, but those who are late talkers and are identified between two and two and a half years of age tend to have lower verbal memories and reading and writing abilities at 13 and 17 years (Rescorla, 2005, 2009). Further, children with language delays are at greater risk for reading, social, and academic difficulties (Tomblin, Zhang, Buckwalter & Catts, 2000). For young children experiencing communication delays, it is important to provide them with opportunities for communication enrichment through preschool programs that facilitate communication and social interaction among young children. Primary care providers should be aware of the value of an enriched preschool program on the development of a late talker.

In Chap. 6, *specific language impairment* is examined which occurs in about 7% of the US population. Specific language impairment (SLI) looks different in different languages; therefore, it is important to ensure appropriate assessment is conducted. Intervention supports are provided as early as possible as there are significant implications for reading comprehension and production and later language learning for children with SLI.

Chapter 7, *Language Learning Disabilities*, highlights the later language learning challenges that children and adolescents with language-based learning disabilities face including written language, reading comprehension, and oral language. In Chap. 8, the focus is on *Speech Sound Disorders and Stuttering*. This chapter emphasizes common speech sound disorders in childhood, including childhood apraxia of cleft lip and palate as well as cerebral palsy. It also includes a description of typical vs. atypical dysfluencies and voice disorders common in childhood.

Hearing Impairment, Chap. 9, emphasizes the importance of assessing and monitoring hearing from newborn hearing screening to considerations for addressing the needs of children with cochlear implants. A discussion of the cultural contexts for deafness and hearing is included. Chapter 10, the *Intellectual Disabilities* chapter, provides the definition for disability, a description of impairments and associated limitations in activity and participation, and the impact of intellectual disabilities on functioning including adaptive behavior.

In the last two chapters, commonly occurring neurodevelopmental disorders with likely social communication impairments are emphasized. Chapter 11 describes attention deficit/hyperactivity disorder (ADHD) and the implications of the disorder for function, learning, and social communication. In the final chapter of the book, Chap. 12, *autism spectrum disorders* is discussed, and the importance of understanding the social communication and social interaction needs of this population is highlighted. Approaches to assessment and providing support are presented for both disorders in their respective chapters.

References

Aram, D. M., & Nation, J. E. (1980). Preschool language disorders and subsequent language and academic difficulties. *Journal of Communication Disorders, 13*, 159–179.

Black, L. I., Vahratian, A., & Hoffman, H. J. (2015). *Communication disorders and use of intervention services among children aged 3–17 years: United States, 2012, NCHS data brief, no 205*. Hyattsville, MD: National Center for Health Statistics.

Center on the Developing Child at Harvard University (2012). The Science of Neglect: The Persistent Absence of Responsive Care Disrupts the Developing Brain: Working Paper No. 12. Retrieved from http://www.developingchild.harvard.edu.

Fernald, A., Marchman, V. A., & Weisleder, A. (2013). SES differences in language processing skill and vocabulary are evident at 18 months. *Developmental Science, 16*, 234–248.

Gillam, R. B., & Marquardt, T. P. (2016). *Communication sciences and disorders: From science to clinical practice*. Burlington, MA: Jones & Bartlett Learning.

Hall, P. K., & Tomblin, J. B. (1978). A follow-up study of children with articulation and language disorders. *Journal of Speech and Hearing Disorders, 43*, 227–241.

Hart, B., & Risley, T. (1995). *Meaningful differences in the everyday experience of young American children*. Baltimore, MD: Paul H. Brookes Publishing.

Lee, V. E., & Burkam, D. T. (2002). Inequality at the starting gate: Social background differences in achievement as children begin school (Executive Summary). Retrieved from http://www.asu.edu/educ/epsl

National Institute on Deafness and Other Communication Disorders (2015a). *Health information*. Retrieved from http://www.nidcd.nih.gov/health/Pages/Default.aspx

National Institute on Deafness and Other Communication Disorders. (2015b). *Statistics on voice, speech and language*. Bethesda, MD: Author Retrieved from http://www.nidcd.nih.gov/health/statistics/Pages/vsl.aspx

Porter, N. (2012). Promotion of pretend play for children with high-functioning autism through the use of circumscribed interests. *Journal of Early Childhood Education, 40*, 161–167.

Rescorla, L. (2005). Age 13 language and reading outcomes in late talking toddlers. *Journal of Speech, Language and Hearing Research, 48*, 459–472.

Rescorla, L. (2009). Age 17 language and reading outcomes in late-talking toddlers: Support for a dimensional perspective on language delay. *Journal of Speech, Language and Hearing Research, 52*, 16–30.

The ASHA Leader. (2015a, August). Almost 8 percent of U.S. children have a communication or swallowing disorder. *20*, 10. doi:https://doi.org/10.1044/leader.NIB1.20082015.10

The ASHA Leader. (2015b, October). National health survey should include dyslexia in communication disorder counts. *20*, 4. doi:https://doi.org/10.1044/leader.IN2.20102015.4

Tomblin, J. B., Zhang, X., Buckwalter, P., & Catts, H. (2000). The association of reading disability, behavioral disorders, and language impairment among second-grade children. *Journal of Child Psychology and Psychiatry, 41*, 473–482.

Walker, D., Greenwood, C., & Hart, B. (1994). Prediction of school outcomes based on early language production and socioeconomic factors. *Child Development, 65*(2), 606–621.

World Health Organization. (2011). *World report on disability*. Geneva, Switzerland: Author Retrieved from http://www.who.int/disabilities/world_report/2011/en/

Chapter 2
An Introduction to Communication Development

Communication, Speech, and Language

The difference between communication, speech, and language is a common point of confusion for many healthcare professionals. Much of the confusion stems from the three terms being used interchangeably in informal discourse. These three features frequently co-occur, but they are, in fact, distinct and separable. The infant who looks to a caregiver and raises her arms to indicate that she would like to be plucked from her highchair is using gestures in the service of *communication*. The 10-month-old who babbles "ba ba ba" while blissfully banging two blocks together is using *speech* but not to communicate a particular meaning. The 1-year-old who exclaims "Mama!" when reunited with his mother is communicating with speech but is also employing *language*.

In describing the nature of typical communicative development, it is first instructive to define communication, speech, and language. Communication is the act of exchanging verbal or nonverbal (as in the use of gestures) information. Speech refers to the production of speech sounds, and it can be linguistic (as in the production of words and sentences) or prelinguistic (as in the babbling of infants). Speech includes:

- Articulation: how speech sounds are made (e.g., the [m] sound is produced by putting the lips together and letting air escape through the nose)
- Phonology: how speech sounds are put together (e.g., children must learn how to produce not only the [s] in "sap" but the [s] in "slap" which is more difficult as it occurs in a consonant cluster)
- Voice: the coordination of breathing and vocal fold vibration to produce sound (also referred to as phonation)
- Fluency: the smooth production of speech, including rhythm (e.g., stuttering is considered a fluency disorder)

P. A. Prelock, T. L. Hutchins, *Clinical Guide to Assessment and Treatment of Communication Disorders*, Best Practices in Child and Adolescent Behavioral Health Care, https://doi.org/10.1007/978-3-319-93203-3_2

By contrast, language is a rule-governed symbolic system that is made up of socially shared rules. Language includes (American Speech, Language, and Hearing Association, 2014):

- Semantics: what words mean (e.g., the word "bug" can refer to an insect or a surveillance device)
- Morphology: how to make new words (e.g., parent, parents, parenting)
- Syntax: how to put words together (e.g., "Mary, the girl next door, loves puppies")
- Pragmatics: the socially appropriate use of language (e.g., understanding sarcasm, using polite constructions like "please" and "thank you," understanding how to take turns and initiate and conclude conversations)

This chapter focuses on typical communication development in infancy, toddlerhood, and early childhood and begins with a description of the patterns of prelinguistic speech and language development seen in infancy. Communicative development in toddlerhood and early childhood is then discussed with an emphasis on articulation, phonological, semantic, and morphosyntactic milestones. Early development of fluency and voice, while important for a fuller understanding of typical development, is not described here. Rather, these domains are explored in subsequent chapters in this book to illustrate the nature of speech or language disorders.

Communicative Development in Infancy: The Prelinguistic Period

The period between birth and 1 year is often referred to as the prelinguistic period. From birth, babies already recognize their mothers' voices. Soon, they also respond to differences between their own language and other languages. Their speech perception becomes more and more language specific throughout this year.

The prelinguistic period also is a time when infants begin to communicate in a variety of ways, but they do all of it without words. During this time infants respond to the language of others, vocalize in different ways, and, later in their first year, are able to use a variety of communicative gestures. Most infants produce their first words around the time of their first birthday, thus marking the end of the prelinguistic period. Prior to first words, however, much has happened to prepare the infant for the successful acquisition of language. We will first describe how different vocalizations develop in infancy.

Getting Ready to Speak

Stages of Vocal Development Infants appear to pass through the same stages of vocal development regardless of the linguistic community in which they are raised. These stages do not have sharp boundaries and tend to overlap with each other. A new stage is marked by the appearance of a new vocalization type, but older vocal behaviors may not disappear until weeks or months after the new one has emerged (Stoel-Gammon & Menn, 2013).

Early Speech Sounds It is in the prelinguistic period that the child's phonological – or speech sound – development begins. At around 6–8 months of age, the child's vocal tract approximates its later adult shape which is necessary for the production of the full range of speech sounds in any given language. These physiological changes coincide with the beginning of the babbling period (Bauman-Waengler, 2009) with phonological production skills that continue to be practiced and refined over the next several years of life.

Vowel sounds are the first speech sounds to be produced and predominate in the early vocal stages described in Table 2.1. In typical development, a limited range of consonant sounds begins to be produced in the babbling stages. The earliest consonants tend to be those that can be produced rather clumsily (e.g., by closing the lips and letting the air escape through the nose as in the [m] sound). The order of speech sound development is largely independent of the child's mother tongue with the most frequent being [h], [d], [b], [m], [t], and [w]. These tend to be followed by [n], [k], [p], and the [j] sound in yoyo (Bauman-Waengler, 2009). Although there is a range of normal developmental timetables, open syllables using vowels (V) and consonants (C) (V, CV, VCV, CVCV) predominate in the later babbling stages, whereas closed syllables (i.e., syllables that end with a C) are relatively rare (Kent & Bauer, 1985).

Prelinguistic Communication Many caregivers notice a qualitative difference in their babies' behavior around the 9th month of life. Prior to this time, babies can

Table 2.1 Stages of vocalization between birth and 1 year

Stage	Description
Stage 1: Reflexive vocalizations (birth–2 months)	Most vocalizations are reflexive (e.g., crying and vegetative sounds like coughing and sneezing). Babies also make some vowel-like sounds
Stage 2: Cooing and laughter (2–4 months)	Rapid growth of the head and neck allows for the production of a wider range of sounds. Infants begin to make comfort-state vocalizations (e.g., cooing); sustained laughter and chuckling appear
Stage 3: Vocal play (4–6 months)	Babies seem to be testing their vocal apparatus. They may produce very loud and very soft sounds (e.g., yells, whispers, squeals), and some babies produce long series of raspberries (trill sounds) and sustained vowels
Stage 4: Canonical babbling (6 months and older)	Babies appear as if they are trying to produce words, but very rhythmically. They use consonant-vowel (CV) sequences to produce reduplicated babbles (strings of identical CV syllables like ba-ba-ba) and variegated syllables (syllable strings with varying CVs like ba-di-gu)
Stage 5: Jargon stage (10 months and older)	Strings of syllables are uttered with a rich variety of stress and intonation patterns that approximate conversational speech; utterances are often accompanied by sustained eye contact and use of gestures

Adapted from Stoel-Gammon and Menn (2013); original in Stark (1986)

move, look around, and smile socially. They take turns vocalizing with caregivers, but there is no indication that they are actually intending to communicate. At around 9 months, however, babies become interesting interaction partners, they are *intentional* in their efforts to gain caregivers' attention and assistance, and they can express a range of communicative functions. This is typically accomplished through looking that is coordinated with gestures (e.g., pointing, reaching) and vocalizing. Different communicative functions have been identified and all of them emerge in typical development before children begin to produce their first words. These functions (adapted from Sachs, 2009) include but are not limited to:

- Requests: gestures and/or vocalizations that are used in service of a goal.
  1. Requests for social interaction: used to attract or maintain someone else's attention (the child who is being ignored may vocalize to get the attention of a caregiver)
  2. Requests for object: used to indicate desire for an object that child cannot reach (e.g., the child looks to partner, looks to object, points to object, and vocalizes to indicate a desired object)
  3. Request for action: used to initiate an action by the partner (e.g., the child lifts hands and vocalizes to indicate she wants to be picked up)
- Rejection: a gesture or vocalization is used to terminate an interaction (e.g., the child vocalizes and turns head away from food that is offered)

The development of intentional communication is also accompanied by a new ability to engage in episodes of joint attention. During joint attention, two people not only attend to an object (e.g., both looking at it), but each also monitors the other's attention to the object. In this way, an interaction partner comes to share attention with another and can be made aware of the contents and attitudes of other minds. Joint attention has been described as having "cosmic" (Bates, 1979) importance for the development of language, and while this ability first emerges in the prelinguistic period, its relation to long-term language outcomes in both populations of children with and without disorders is well-documented.

Communicative Development: Toddlerhood and Early Childhood

Speech

Speech Sound Production As noted above, the first speech sounds are vowel sounds. These are followed by a limited set of consonants which emerges in the babbling stages and is relatively easy to produce. As children move into toddlerhood, their repertoire of consonant sounds continues to develop and more challenging sounds begin to appear. These more challenging sounds are often from a class of sounds that are vowel-like (liquid, e.g., [l]). Other challenging sounds are produced by forcing air through a narrow space between articulators (fricative, e.g., [s]) or by stopping air briefly before forcing it through a narrow space (affricate, e.g., "ch"). These more challenging sounds may take several years to master, and they vary from language to language. The average age estimates for customary production (i.e., the point when the child is producing a sound correctly more often than he/she misarticulates or omits the sound) of English consonants are presented in Fig. 2.1. Of course, when children are learning to produce the individual speech sounds that comprise their native tongue, they are really working with larger segments of speech like consonant clusters (blends), syllables, and words. Thus, it is also important to also consider children's development of speech structures. These, too, vary from language to language. For example, in English, first words are primarily one syllable long; in some other languages, one-syllable words are actually rare, and children's first words are typically two or more syllables long.

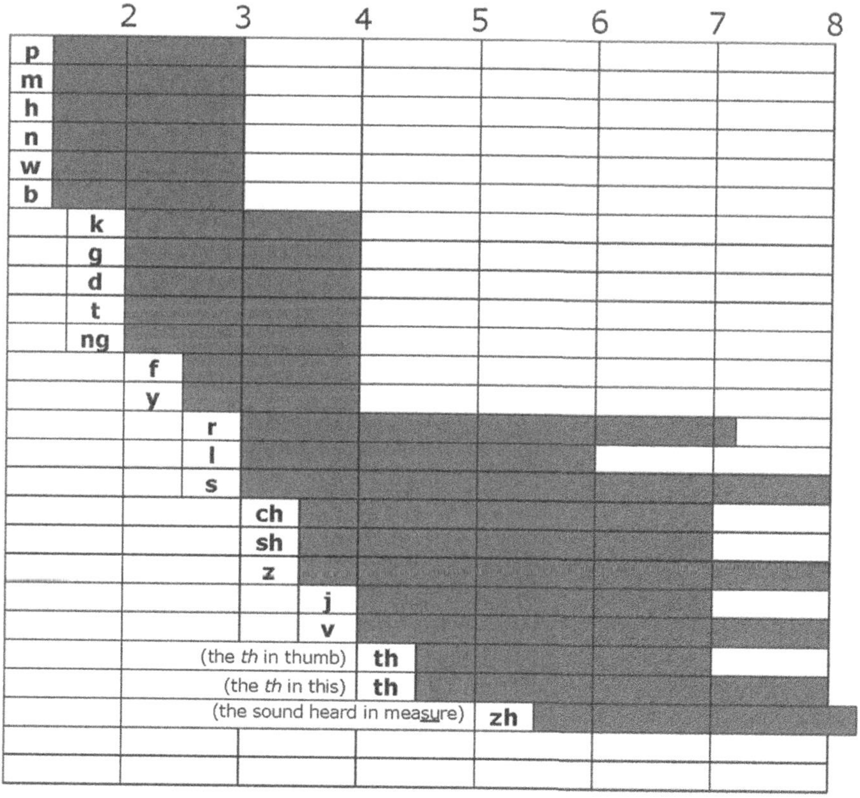

Fig. 2.1 Age ranges of typical consonant development. (Average age estimates and upper age limits of customary English consonant production. The solid bar corresponding to each sound starts at the median age of customary articulation; it stops at age level at which 90% of all children are producing the sound. From Sander (1972))

Intelligibility Intelligibility refers to the clarity of speech and the amount of a speaker's output that a listener can readily understand. It is the most reliable aspect of a child's speech for caregivers to report. The intelligibility of young children is affected by speaking context (e.g., it tends to be higher in single words compared to connected speech) as well as the listener's experience with the child. Primary caregivers may be more tuned-in to their children's speech production and often understand more of the child's speech than can strangers or even familiar adults. It is well-established that in typical development, increases in chronological age are associated with higher degrees of intelligibility. Generally accepted norms hold that by age 2 years, children should be about 50% intelligible (defined as the percent of words understood in connected speech); that by age 3 years, children should be about 75% intelligible; and that by age 4 years, children should be 100% intelligible (Coplan & Gleason, 1988). In fact, for children 4 years or older, intelligibility less than 66% (two standard deviations below the mean) may be considered a potential indicator of speech difficulty (Gordon-Brannan & Hodson, 2000).

Phonology The most important function of speech sounds is to differentiate words. If every word a child attempts sounds like "ba," adults will not be able to understand what she is trying to say. Contrastive consonants and vowels, called "phonemes" when they have this function, differentiate words. For example, /b/ and /d/ differentiate "bad" from "dad" in English; similarly, /b/ and /d/ differentiate "beau" ("handsome," pronounced as [bo]) from "d'eau" ("some water," pronounced as [do]) in French. If a child substitutes [b] for /d/ or vice versa, confusion will result. Various word structures also differentiate words, depending on the rules of the language. For example, the number of syllables differentiates "d'eau" from "dodo" – "sleep," pronounced as [dodo] – in French and "boo" (said to surprise someone) from "boo-boo" (sore) in English. A final consonant differentiates "boo" from "boot" in English; an /l/ in the initial consonant cluster (blend) differentiates "plain," "ground," from "pain" – "bread" in French. Producing these structures correctly ensures listener understanding.

Various error patterns interfere with these contrastive functions of consonants, vowels, and word structures during development. These error patterns, often called "phonological processes," describe what typically developing children do in their early speech productions to simplify the standard adult forms (Shipley & McAfee, 2009). For example, children will often simplify a consonant cluster (e.g., the [bl] sound in "block") by dropping one of the consonants (e.g., "bock") or replacing the cluster with a different single consonant (e.g., "wock"). They may also replace harder consonant sounds produced at the back of the mouth (e.g., /k/) with easier ones produced near the front of the mouth (e.g., [t] so "kill" becomes "till") in a process called "fronting."

Numerous phonological processes are common in the speech production of children. Some of the more common processes in the speech of English-learning children are summarized in Table 2.2. However, it is important to note that different processes are common in different languages. For example, if an English-speaking child over the age of 30 months continues to omit initial consonants, that is a "red flag" for a possible disorder; the process of "initial consonant deletion" is rare in

Table 2.2 Description of common phonological processes seen in typical English development

Processes disappearing by age 3 years	Processes persisting beyond age 3 years
Unstressed syllable deletion: deletion of an unstressed syllable (e.g., "telephone" ➔ "tephone"; "pajamas" ➔ "jammas")	*Consonant cluster reduction*: simplifying a cluster by dropping one consonant sound or replacing the cluster with a different single consonant sound (e.g., "block" ➔ "bock"; "mask" ➔ "mack")
Final consonant deletion: deletion of a final consonant ("bat" ➔ "ba"; "rode" ➔ "ro")	*Gliding*: substituting a glide sound for a liquid sound (e.g., "run" ➔ "wun"; "yellow" ➔ "yewow")
Reduplication: repetition of a complete or incomplete syllable ("water" ➔ "wawa"; "soap" ➔ "soso")	*Epenthesis*: insertion of a phoneme (e.g., "black" ➔ "belack"; "color" ➔ "cluller")
Doubling: repetition of a word (e.g., "go" ➔ "go go"; "dad" ➔ "dada")	*Stopping*: substituting a stop for a fricative or affricate ("sun" ➔ "tun"; "batch" ➔ "bat")
Diminutization: addition of "eee" sound at the end of a word (e.g., "horse" ➔ "horsie"; "pig" ➔ "piggy")	*Vocalization*: substituting a vowel for a liquid in the final position (e.g., "better" ➔ "betto"; "fiddle" ➔ "fiddo")

Adapted from Stoel-Gammon and Dunn (1985), Shipley and McAfee (2009)

typically developing children learning that language. However, this process is quite common in a variety of other languages, including French, Welsh, and Japanese; it is not a cause for concern until later ages. Generally speaking, English-learning children are expected to outgrow the phonological processes appearing on the left-hand side of the table by age 3 (Stoel-Gammon & Dunn, 1985). The phonological processes on the right-hand side of the table tend to persist beyond age 3, but *all* phonological processes are expected to be resolved by age 8 in English-speaking children (Stoel-Gammon & Dunn, 1985). Of course, when a child uses many different processes or uses processes that are not common during speech acquisition, the child's intelligibility is likely to be reduced.

Receptive and Expressive Language

When describing language development, it is important to make a distinction between receptive and expressive language. Receptive language refers to language (across all of the semantic, morphology, syntax, and pragmatic domains) that the child understands, whereas expressive language refers to the language that the child can produce. As we will see, a general pattern in typical language development is that receptive skills tend to precede and outstrip expressive skills across domains. In this section, we will identify timetables for major developmental milestones and describe the content of children's early vocabularies and morphosyntactic constructions.

Semantics Semantic development describes the process of how children come to learn the meanings of words. Children begin to produce their first words around their first birthday (with 8–16 months often identified as the wider range of normal), but children's receptive vocabulary emerges earlier and tends to accompany the developments of intentional communication and joint attention that were described above. Words tend to be added, slowly at first and at an accelerated rate later on. More specifically, when children achieve an approximate 50-word productive vocabulary, which tends to be around 18 months, many of them experience a kind of vocabulary explosion or "word spurt." This word spurt has been described as a rapid increase in the number of words that children know and use. Although several studies have documented the word spurt, it is also clear that not all children show dramatic change and that the rate of word acquisition varies greatly across children as they approach age 2 years (Ganger & Brent, 2004).

Whether the trend is gradual or abrupt, the rate at which children learn words is prodigious. One reason for this is that children appear to need neither explicit information about (e.g., "This is a cup" while pointing to a cup) nor frequent experience with a word to learn or remember something about it (Carey & Bartlett, 1978). For example, weeks after a child hears "Hand me the *molby* shoe; not the blue shoe, the *molby* shoe" in an experiment, he is likely able to demonstrate his understanding that *molby* is a color term. Although children can acquire word meanings (partial or complete) with a single exposure, it is also true that more frequent exposure to a word is associated with enhanced semantic development and this seems to be particularly important for the acquisition of meanings that are more abstract (e.g., "devotion") or linguistically complex (e.g., verbs like "teach" and "learn") (Gropen, Pinker, Hollander, & Goldberg, 1991).

The first words of children are often tied to the situational context. For example, a child may say "duck" in reference to a rubber duck while playing in the bathtub but does not use the word to refer to the same rubber duck if it is in the bedroom. Similarly the child may not apply the label "duck" when confronted with ducks appearing in picture books or when seeing them in real life. This kind of context-bound usage is part of typical language development and is one example of "underextension." The term underextension refers to the use of a word in a way that does not include its full range of meaning (e.g., assuming that the word "cat" only refers to the family cat). It soon disappears as children learn to unhinge a word from the setting.

By contrast, in overextensions, the child uses a word in a broader context than is permissible in adult usage (e.g., calling all men "daddy"). It was once thought that overextensions *only* reflected incomplete or incorrect concept formation (i.e., the child is failing to understand those features that "daddy" and "man" share and do not share). However, children may also produce overextensions because of recall difficulties or because they lack the proper label for a concept and are using the word that they know with the most similar meaning (Gelman, Croft, Fu, Clasuner, & Gottfried, 1998; Hoek, Ingram, & Gibson, 1986). Underextensions and overextensions are common in the language of 1- and 2-year-olds and account for nearly one third of their productive vocabularies (Clark, 1995). They are far less frequent in the output of older children.

With regard to content, children's early vocabularies tend to be dominated by nouns. This is a relatively robust finding across languages (see Bornstein, Cote,

Table 2.3 Children's early vocabularies: examples from children younger than 20 months

Sound effects	Woof, yum-yum, meow, ruff-ruff
Food and drink	Apple, banana, juice, water, cookie
Animals	Bear, dog, cat, horse, duck, kitty
Body parts and clothing	Diaper, ear, eye, mouth, nose, teeth, pajamas
House and outdoors	Bed, chair, cup, blanket, spoon, flower, tree
People	Baby, daddy, mommy, grandma
Toys and vehicles	Ball, balloon, bike, boat, book, bubbles
Actions	Down, eat, go, sit, up
Games and routines	Bath, bye, hi, night-night, no, peek-a-boo, please, thank you
Adjectives and descriptive	All gone, cold, dirty, hot

Adapted from Uccelli and Pan (2013)

Maital, Painter, & Park, 2004) that may be due to the fact that nouns tend to be less linguistically complex compared to words from other grammatical classes (e.g., verbs). Words that make up children's early vocabularies also tend to reflect a limited number of semantic classes and often refer to things that are important in the child's life. Examples of words produced by children under 20 months of age are offered in Table 2.3.

Morphosyntax Morphology refers to rules for building words (e.g., walk + ed ➔ past tense of walk), whereas syntax refers to rules for building sentences (e.g., a sentence is composed of a noun phrase "the cat" + a verb phrase "ran fast"). Thus, morphosyntactic development describes the process of how children begin to build words and to combine them in a systematic way. First words are uttered in isolation and referred to as "holophrases." A holophrase is a single word that is intended to express a complete thought (e.g., a child who says "cat" may intend to mean "look at the cat"). Because advances in semantic development closely parallel advances in syntactic development, it is not surprising that around 18 months – when children are experiencing significant growth in vocabulary – they also begin to produce two-word combinations (e.g., "my doggie"). Prior to this, however, children know much more about the rules of their language than their use of two-word combinations suggests. In fact, it has been demonstrated that as young as 17 months of age, children understand the difference between utterances like "the cow kicked the horse" and "the horse kicked the cow" (Hirsh-Pasek & Golinkoff, 1987, 1993). This understanding is rooted in an impressive syntactic knowledge where the child must identify the doer (subject) and receiver (direct object) of an action on the basis of word position in a sentence. Thus, as it was with semantic development, receptive syntactic skills generally precede and outstrip a child's expressive skills.

Nonetheless, the emergence of two-word combinations is an important milestone that allows children to communicate about a wide range of topics. These topics are captured by the term "semantic relations" to highlight the relational meaning between words. Examples of common semantic relations found in the two-word utterances of 14–24-month-olds are presented in Table 2.4.

Table 2.4 Common semantic relations in the language of 14–22-month-olds

Relation	Example
Agent + action	Mommy come; daddy sit
Action + object	Drive car; eat grape
Agent + object	Mommy book; baby sock
Action + location	Go park; sit chair
Entity + location	Cup table; toy floor
Possessor + possession	My teddy; mommy dress
Entity + attribute	Box shiny; crayon big
Demonstrative + entity	That money; this telephone
Disappearance/nonexistence	All gone/no shoe
Recurrence	More juice
Rejection	No juice (I don't want use)
Denial	Not tired

Adapted from Zukowski (2013)

Table 2.5 Order of acquisition of 14 grammatical morphemes (Brown, 1973)

Rank	Morphological feature	Example	Age of mastery (in months)
1	Present progressive -ing	Daddy sing<u>ing</u>	19–28
2	In	Key <u>in</u> cup	27–30
3	on	Ball <u>on</u> bed	27–33
4	Regular plural -s	Two cat<u>s</u>	27–33
5	Irregular past tense	Mommy <u>fell</u>	25–46
6	Possessive -s	Mommy'<u>s</u> car	26–40
7	Uncontractible copula	She <u>is</u> (in response to: who is nice?)	28–46
8	Articles	I got <u>a</u> dog. I got <u>the</u> ball	28–46
9	Regular past tense -ed	Daddy walk<u>ed</u>	26–48
10	Regular third person -s	Mommy walk<u>s</u>	28–50
11	Irregular third person	Daddy <u>has</u> a ball	28–50
12	Uncontractible auxiliary	She <u>might</u> go	29–48
13	Contractible copula	He'<u>s</u> happy	29–49
14	Contractible auxiliary	I'<u>d</u> like that	30–50

Three-word utterances may also occur toward the end of the child's second year; however, certain types of words (e.g., a, the, in, on) and morphemes (e.g., past tense -ed, plural -s, present progressive -ing in English) tend to be missing. Because several common words and morphemes are usually absent, the multi-word utterances of very young children can sound like the sentences produced in a telegram (e.g., "give juice" for "give me the juice" or "mommy cup" for "mommy's cup). This "telegraphic speech" (Brown & Fraser, 1963) has been documented in a number of different languages (Hoff, 2001).

Between 24 and 30 months, however, the once-absent words and morphemes begin to emerge, and they do so in a fairly predictable order. The order described here (see Table 2.5) is based on English morphemes; it is important to note that the structure of the language that the child is learning can influence the sequence and

Table 2.6 Summary of phonological, semantic, and syntactic milestones of early communicative development in English

Typical age	Pragmatics	Phonology	Semantics	Syntax
0–8 mo.	Caregivers attribute intent to child's actions and vocalizations	0–2 mo – vegetative sounds 2–4 mo – cooing, laughing 4–6 mo – vocal play, sustained vowels 6–10 mo – canonical and reduplicated babbling		
8–12 mo.	Joint attention and communicative intent emerges. Communicative functions such as: Request for social interaction Requesting for object Request for action Rejection	Jargon and babble with intonation contours of the language being learned	Understanding 3–50 words First words used for names of familiar people and objects, communicative games, and routines; talk about disappearance, recurrence	
12–18 mo.	Frequency of communicative intent is ~ 5 per 1 min of free play	First 50 words: Most often have CV shape Use same consonants used in early babbling Use of reduplication, unstressed syllable deletion, consonant cluster reduction, and final consonant deletion	Average expressive vocabulary of 50–100 words at 18 mo Semantic roles expressed in one-word speech include agent, action, object, location, possession, rejection, disappearance, nonexistence, denial	
18–24 mo.	Frequency of communicative intent is ~ 7.5 per 1 min of free play New communicative intents include: Requesting information Answering questions	By 24 mo, 9–10 initial and 5–6 final consonants are used Speech is 50% intelligible 70% of consonants are correct CVC and two syllable words emerge	Average expressive vocabulary of 200–300 words at 24 mo Understand two-word relations similar to those expressed which include agent-action, agent-object, action-object, action-location, entity-location, possessor-possession, demonstrative-entity, attribute-entity	Two-word utterances emerge Word order is consistent Utterances are "telegraphic" with few grammatical markers

(continued)

Table 2.6 (continued)

Typical age	Pragmatics	Phonology	Semantics	Syntax
24–30 mo.	New communicative intents include: Symbolic play Talk about absent objects Misrepresenting reality (lies, teases)	Awareness of rhyme emerges	Understanding and use of questions about objects (what), people (who), basic events (what x doing?; where x going?)	Grammatical morphemes emerge: -ing, in, on, plural /s/ Use of no, not, can't, don't Questions formed with rising intonation only
30–36 mo.	Child able to continue a topic ~ 50% of the time Topics are continued by adding new information	Speech is 75% intelligible at 36 mo Ability to produce rhyme emerges	Use and understanding of "why" questions	Present tense auxiliaries appear (can, will) "Be" verbs used inconsistently Overregularization of past tense (e.g., hitted, drawed)
36–42 mo.	More flexibility in requesting including "Can you…?" and "Would you…?" constructions	Use of reduplication, unstressed syllable, deletion, and final consonant deletion is less common	Understanding of basic color terms Use and understanding of basic kinship terms	First embedded sentences appear; irregular past tense (e.g., hit, drew), articles (a, the), and possessive -s (e.g., Mary's) emerge
42–48 mo.	New communicative functions include: Reporting on past events Predicting Reasoning Expressing empathy Creating imaginary roles	Use of consonant cluster reduction decreases	Use and understanding of "when" and" how" questions Understanding of words for basic shapes (circle, square, triangle) Use and understanding of basic vocabulary (big, small) Use of conjunctions and because to conjoin sentences	Complex sentence types emerge including: Full prepositional phrase (e.g., The girl *in white shirt* drank juice) Wh-clauses (e.g., The girl *with the book* drank juice) Simple infinitives (e.g., She wants *to read* a book)

Table 2.6 (continued)

Typical age	Pragmatics	Phonology	Semantics	Syntax
48–60 mo.	Hints that do not mention the intention of the request ("Those smell good!") Child more able to address requests for clarification	Speech is 100% intelligible Ability to segment words into syllable emerges Use of most phonological processes stops; errors on more difficult consonants may persist, especially in more complex structures (such as consonant clusters)	Knowledge of letter names and sounds emerges Knowledge of numbers and counting emerges Use of conjunctions when, so, because, if	All basic sentence forms acquired Later developing forms emerge including: "Be" verbs Regular past Third person -s (He hits the ball)

Adapted from Paul and Norbury (2012); data from Chapman (2000), Miller (1981) Weiss, Gordon and Lilywhite (1987) developmental timetables associated with morphosyntactic development. For instance, children acquiring Turkish have been reported to produce inflected morphemes (e.g., plural forms) before they begin to combine words (Aksu-Koc & Slobin, 1985).

Early sentences tend to be in the affirmative and declarative form (e.g., "The cat is black"), but as the child adds to her morphemic repertoire, she is able to form more advanced sentence types. Although children find ways to negate and ask questions before they have acquired all the necessary words (e.g., they can ask a question by saying "My cup?" with rising intonation), the adult forms require morphemes (e.g., auxiliary verbs like "will," "would") in English. Once these words are mastered, the forms of children's negative statements and questions change (Hoff, 2001). After the development of morphemes and different sentence forms is underway, the next morphosyntactic development is the appearance of sentences that contain more than one clause (Hoff, 2001). There are many different types of complex sentences, and they vary in terms of their general developmental timetables. A summary of the major phonological, semantic, and morphosyntacic milestones, including examples of complex sentence types, is presented in Table 2.6.

References

Aksu-Koc, A. A., & Slobin, D. I. (1985). The acquisition of Turkish. In D. I. Slobin (Ed.), *The crosslinguistic study of language acquisition* (Vol. 1. The data, pp. 839–880). Hillsdale, NJ: Erlbaum.

American Speech, Language, and Hearing Association. (2014). What is language? What is speech? Retrieved January 6, 2014 from http://www.asha.org/public/speech/development/language_speech.htm

Bates, E. (1979). *The emergence of symbols: Cognition and communication in infancy*. New York: Academic Press.

Bauman-Waengler, J. (2009). *Introduction to phonetics and phonology: From concepts to transcription*. New York: Pearson.

Bornstein, M., Cote, L., Maital, S., Painter, K., & Park, S. (2004). Crosslinguistic analysis of vocabulary in young children: Spanish, Dutch, French, Hebrew, Italian, Korean, and American English. *Child Development, 75*, 1115–1139.

Brown, R. (1973). *A first language: The early stages*. Cambridge, MA: Harvard University Press.

Brown, R., & Fraser, C. (1963). The acquisition of syntax. In C. N. Cofer & B. S. Musgrave (Eds.), *Verbal behavior and learning* (pp. 158–196). New York: McGraw-Hill.

Carey, S., & Bartlett, E. (1978). Acquiring a single new word. *Papers and Reports on Child Language Development, 15*, 17–29.

Chapman, R. (2000). Children's language learning.: An interactionist perspective. *Journal of Child Psychology and Psychiatry, 41*, 33–54.

Clark, E. (1995). *The lexicon in acquisition*. Cambridge, UK: Cambridge University Press.

Coplan, J., & Gleason, J. (1988). Unclear speech: Recognition and significance of unintelligible speech in preschool children. *Pediatrics, 82*(3), 447–452.

Ganger, J., & Brent, M. (2004). Reexamining the vocabulary spurt. *Developmental Psychology, 40*, 621–632.

Gelman, S., Croft, W., Fu, P., Clausner, T., & Gottfried, G. (1998). Why is a pomegranate an apple? The role of shape, taxonomic relatedness, and prior lexical knowledge in children's overextensions of apple and dog. *Journal of Child Language, 25*, 267–291.

Gordon-Brannan, M., & Hodson, B. W. (2000). Intelligibility/severity measurements of prekindergarten children's speech. *American Journal of Speech Language Pathology, 9*(2), 141–150.

Gropen, J., Pinker, S., Hollander, M., & Goldberg, R. (1991). Syntax and semantics in the acquisition of locative verbs. *Journal of Child Language, 18*(1), 115–151.

Hirsh-Pasek, K., & Golinkoff, R. M. (1987). The eyes have it: Lexical and syntactic comprehension in a new paradigm. *Journal of Child Language, 14*, 23–45.

Hirsh-Pasek, K., & Golinkoff, R. M. (1993). Skeletal supports for grammatical learning: What the infant brings to the language learning task. In C. K. Rovee-Collier (Ed.), *Advances in Infancy Research* (Vol. 8, pp. 299–338). Norwood, NJ: Ablex.

Hoek, D., Ingram, D., & Gibson, D. (1986). Some possible causes of children's early word overextensions. *Journal of Child Language, 13*, 477–494.

Hoff, E. (2001). *Language development* (2nd ed.). Stamford, CT: Wadsworth.

Kent, R. D., & Bauer, H. R. (1985). Vocalizations of one-year-olds. *Journal of Child Language, 13*, 491–526.

Miller, J. (1981). *Assessing language production in children*. Boston, MA: Allyn & Bacon.

Paul, R., & Norbury, C. (2012). *Language disorders: From infancy through adolescence* (4th ed.). St. Louis, MO: Elsevier.

Sachs, J. (2009). Communication development in infancy. In J. Berko Gleason & N. Bernstein Ratner (Eds.), *The development of language* (pp. 37–57). New York: Pearson.

Sander, E. K. (1972). When are speech sounds learned? *Journal of Speech and Hearing Disorders, 37*, 55–63.

Shipley, K. G., & McAfee, J. G. (2009). *Assessment in speech-language pathology* (4th ed.). Clifton Park, NY: Delmar Cengage Learning.

Stark, R. (1986). Prespeech segmental feature development. In P. Fletcher & M. Garman (Eds.), *Language acquisition: Studies in first language development* (pp. 149–173). Cambridge, UK: Cambridge University Press.

Stoel-Gammon, C., & Menn, L. (2013). Phonological development: Learning sounds and sound patterns. In J. Berko Gleason & N. Bernstein Ratner (Eds.), *The development of language* (pp. 52–88). New York: Pearson.

Stoel-Gammon, D., & Dunn, D. (1985). *Normal and disordered phonology in children*. Austin, TX: Pro-Ed.

Uccelli, P., & Pan, B. (2013). Semantic development: Learning the meaning of words. In J. Berko Gleason & N. Bernstein Ratner (Eds.), *The development of language* (pp. 89–119). New York: Pearson.

Weiss, C. E., Gordon, M.E., & Lillywhite, H.S. (1987). *Clinical management of articulatory and phonologic disorders*. Netherlands: Wolters Kluwer.

Zukowski, A. (2013). Putting words together: Morphology and syntax in the preschool years. In J. Berko Gleason & N. Bernstein Ratner (Eds.), *The development of language* (pp. 120–162). New York: Pearson.

Chapter 3
Approaches to the Screening and Identification of Communication Disorders

Introduction

Screening and identification (i.e., diagnosis) are closely related. Screening determines whether an individual should be examined more closely for the possible presence of a disorder. It is important in the realm of public health, particularly for communication disorders, which constitute an important problem, are relatively common, and have readily available treatments. Identification confirms or disconfirms the presence of a disorder that may have been suspected by referral sources or uncovered through a screening procedure (McCauley, 2001).

Although communication disorders, or more specifically speech and language disorders, are the most common childhood disabilities, they are the least well-detected, particularly in primary care settings (Prelock, Hutchins, & Glascoe, 2008). Speech and language deficits affect about 1 in 12 preschool children (or 5–8%), and the consequences of untreated communication problems are significant. They can lead to behavioral challenges, mental health problems, reading difficulties, academic failure, and difficulty establishing successful social relationships (Prelock et al., 2008). In light of the positive consequences of early identification, our aim must be to prevent, detect, and intervene with children with communication disorders as early as possible.

Several screening and identification procedures for specific communication disorders exist and are described in the appropriate chapters in this volume. This chapter will first identify some popular "broadband" measures that are used to screen for problems across different areas of development. These screens are commonly used by pediatricians and other primary care providers including family practice physicians and family nurse practitioners at well-child visits as well as NICU settings for surveillance of potential problems in language, motor, (pre-) academics, self-help, behavior, and social and emotional health. Commonly used measures are presented in Table 3.1.

P. A. Prelock, T. L. Hutchins, *Clinical Guide to Assessment and Treatment of Communication Disorders*, Best Practices in Child and Adolescent Behavioral Health Care, https://doi.org/10.1007/978-3-319-93203-3_3

Table 3.1 Popular broadband measures that include a language component

Scale name (abbreviation)	Age range	Administration	Comment
Ages and Stages Questionnaire (3rd ed.) (ASQ-3; Squires, Potter, & Bricker, 2014)	1–66 months	10–15 min	Items focus on self-regulation, compliance, communication, adaptive functioning, autonomy, affect, and interaction with people. Readily available in multiple languages
Brigance (r) Infant and Toddler Screen – II (Brigance & Glascoe, 2002)	Infant screen: Birth–11 months Toddler screen: 12–23 months	15 min	Language portion screens receptive and expressive vocabulary and syntax
Brigance (r) Early Preschool Screen – II (Brigance & Glascoe, 2005)	2 years–2 years, 11 months	15 min	Language portion screens articulation, fluency, morphosyntax, expressive vocabulary, and reading readiness
Denver Developmental Screening Test (Denver-II; Frankenburg et al., 1992)	Birth–6 years	10–15 min	Uses both parent and direct observation to tap articulation and receptive and expressive vocabulary, syntax. Popular and easily administered but suffers from a number of psychometric weaknesses
Parents' Evaluation of Developmental Status (PEDS; Glascoe, 1998)	Birth–8 years		Language items focus on expressive and receptive language. Readily available in a large number of languages (see http://www.pedstest.com/Translations/PEDSinOtherLanguages.aspx)

Several screens and diagnostic tools specific to language also exist. Some measures (what we term "comprehensive language measures") are designed to detect problems across language domains. The areas assessed by comprehensive language measures often include many or all of the following, although some are restricted to only the first two areas:

- Receptive and expressive semantic (i.e., vocabulary) development
- Receptive and expressive morphosyntactic development (i.e., putting words and sentences together)
- Articulation (i.e., making speech sounds)
- Phonology (i.e., using speech sounds in systematically organized manner)
- Fluency (i.e., smoothness and flow of speech sounds)
- Cognitive processes like working memory that are important to the development of language
- Metalinguistic processes like rhyming and word segmentation that are important for language and literacy development and academic success

A short list of popular comprehensive language screens is presented in Table 3.2. It is important to note, however, that most of the identification (i.e., diagnostic) measures identified in the subsequent table (Table 3.3) are explicitly offered not only as tools that can aid in identification but as screening tools as well.

Of course, some language measures (what we term "specific domain measures") are commonly used as part of a larger assessment battery to provide a more detailed portrait of functioning when there is concern in a particular language area (e.g.,

Table 3.2 Popular comprehensive language measures: screening instruments

Scale name (abbreviation)	Age range	Administration	Comment
Clinical Evaluation of Language Fundamentals-5 Screening (CELF-5 Screening Test; Semel, Wiig, & Secord, 2013)	5 years–21 years, 11 months	15 min	Screens for receptive and expressive language including semantics, grammar, recall, and ability to follow directions; designed for use with CELF-5 (described below)
Fluharty-2 (Fluharty, 2001)	3 years–6 years, 11 months	10 min	Screens for receptive and expressive language including semantics, grammar, articulation, recall, and ability to sequence events; yields global language quotient
The Language Development Survey (LDS, Rescorla, 1989)	18–35 months	10–15 min	Parent informant measure of expressive vocabulary and syntax as well as risk factors for language delay for ages 18–35 months. The LDS can be completed for older children with language delays for comparison with norms up to 35 months

Table 3.3 Popular comprehensive language measures: identification instruments

Scale name (abbreviation)	Age range	Administration	Comment
Comprehensive Assessment of Spoken Language (CASL; Carrow-Woolfolk, 1999) (CASL-2; Carrow-Woolfold, 2017)	3–21 years	5–10 min for subtests; 45 min for core language compositie	Broadband measure designed to tap basic concepts, semantics, syntax, morphology, pragmatics, and memory
Clinical Evaluation of Language Fundamentals, 5th ed. (CELF-5; Semel, Wiig, & Secord, 2013)	5–21 years	30–45 min	Well-validated broadband measure designed to tap basic concepts, semantics, syntax, morphology, pragmatics, phonological awareness, and memory
Early Language Milestone Scale, 2nd ed. (ELMS-2; Coplan, 1993)	Birth–36 months for language development 18–48 months for intelligibility	1–10 min	43-item scale divided into 3 domains: auditory expressive (e.g., babbling, first words, two-word combinations), auditory receptive (e.g., orienting to voice, inhibiting to "no"), and visual (e.g., smiling, imitating gestures). Items elicited through parent history, direct testing, or incidental observation
Test of Early Language Development, 3rd ed. (TELD-3; Hresko, Reid, & Hammill, 1999)	2 years–7 years, 11 months	15–40 min	Designed to assess early development of spoken language in the areas of receptive and expressive language, syntax, and semantics. Can be used as a screen or identification tool
Test of Language Development: Preschool, 4th ed. (TOLD-P4; Newcomer & Hammill, 2008)	4 years–8 years, 11 months	30–60 min	Test of receptive/expressive vocabulary, morphosyntax, and articulation/phonology. Results of subtests can be combined to yield scores for the major dimensions of semantics and grammar; listening, organizing, and speaking; and overall language ability

articulation or semantic development). Specific domain measures generally direct their focus on either vocabulary and/or morphosyntax (Table 3.4) or articulation and phonology (Table 3.5).

Screening and Referral

Early screening can result in treatment, and sometimes prevention, of language problems associated with a diverse set of neurobiological and psychosocial risk factors. Once speech-language impairment is suspected, referral to early

Table 3.4 Popular specific domain measures: vocabulary or grammar development

Scale name (abbreviation)	Age range	Administration	Comment
Expressive One-Word Picture Vocabulary Test-4th ed. (EOWPVT-4; Brownell, 2010a)	2 years–70+ years	15–25 min	Co-normed with the *Receptive One-Word Picture Vocabulary Test*; assesses expressive vocabulary of objects, actions, and concepts; available in Spanish-Bilingual version
Receptive One-Word Picture Vocabulary Test-4th ed. (ROWPVT-4; Brownell, 2010b)	2 years–70+ years	15–25 min	Co-normed with the *Expressive One-Word Picture Vocabulary Test*; assesses receptive vocabulary of objects, actions, and concepts; available in Spanish-Bilingual version
Expressive Vocabulary Test (2nd ed.) (EVT-2; Williams, 2007)	2 years, 6 months–90+ years	10–20 min	Co-normed with the *Receptive One-Word Picture Vocabulary Test*; assesses expressive vocabulary a variety in terms of parts of speech and content
MacArthur-Bates Communicative Development Inventories (CDIs; Fenson et al., 2007)	CDI: Words and gestures: 8–18 months CDI: Words and sentences: 16–30 months	Each of 2 forms takes between 10 and 20 min to complete	Well-validated parent-informant measures: *Words and Gestures* taps emerging receptive and expressive vocabulary and the use of communicative or symbolic gestures; *Words and Sentences* measures expressive vocabulary and grammar. Available in a variety of languages; many of which have supporting normative data (see http://mb-cdi.stanford.edu/adaptations_ol.htm)
Peabody Picture Vocabulary Test (4th ed.) (PPVT-4; Dunn & Dunn, 2007)	2 years, 6 months–90+ years	10–15 min	Well-validated measure of receptive vocabulary; available in a variety of English dialects and other language translations
Structured Photographic Expressive Language Test-Preschool 2nd ed. (SPELT-P2; Dawson et al., 2005)	3 years–5 years, 11 months	20 min	Designed as a test of grammar (i.e., morphosyntax) development; guidance provided for testing children who speak African American English; would benefit from more development

Table 3.5 Popular specific domain measures: Articulation and phonology

Scale name (abbreviation)	Age range	Administration	Comment
Arizona Articulation Proficiency Scale, 3rd ed. (Arizona-3; Fudala, 2000)	1 year, 5 months–18 years	3 min	Tests single-word articulation of consonants and vowels; can help quantify degree of intelligibility
Bankson Bernthal Test of Phonology (BBTOP; Bankson & Bernthal, 1990)	3 years–9 years	10–15 min	Well-validated test of articulation and phonology
Clinical Assessment of Articulation and Phonology-2nd. ed. (CAAP-2; Secord & Donahue, 2013)	2.6 years–11.11 years	15–20 min	Designed to sample children's productions of singleton consonants and consonant clusters in mono- and multisyllabic words and compare production accuracy in words and connected speech. Not an ideal instrument for use in treatment planning
Comprehensive Test of Phonological Processes -2nd ed. (CTOPP-2; Wagner, Torgesen, Rashotte, & Pearson, 2013)	5 years–25 years	30 min	Offered as a test of types of phonological processing that are related to reading (e.g., blending words, isolating sounds, nonword repetition)
Goldman-Fristoe Test of Articulation -3rd ed. (GTFA-3; Goldman & Fristoe, 2015)	2 years–21 years, 11 months	5–15 min	Test of articulation; may be less appropriate when used with nonstandard English speakers on nonstandard English; tips for use in telepractice
Hodson Assessment of Phonological Patterns, 3rd ed. (HAPP-3; Hodson, 2004)	3 years–8 years	15–20 min	Test of phonological patterns; used as a screen or identification tool to assess phonological error patterns of children who have unintelligible speech
Test of Phonological Awareness, 2nd ed.: PLUS (TOPA-2+, Torgessen & Bryant, 2004)	5 years–8 years	15–30 min	Tests awareness of sound patterns including children's ability to isolate individual speech sounds and their knowledge of relationships between letters and phonemes

intervention is the first step, including intervention by speech-language pathologists. Speech-language pathologists and other early interventionists can provide activities within home and school or after-school tutoring programs to support development and provide progress monitoring (Prelock, Gulbronson, Hutchins, Green, & Glascoe, 2013).

References

Bankson, N., & Bernthal, J. (1990). *Bankson-Bernthal test of phonology*. Austin, TX: Pro-Ed.

Brigance, A., & Glascoe, F. (2005). *Brigance (r) early preschool screen – II*. North Billerica, MA: Curriculum Associates.

Brigance, A., & Glascoe, F. (2002). *Brigance (r) infant and toddler screen – II*. North Billerica, MA: Curriculum Associates.

Carrow-Woolfolk, E. (1999). *Comprehensive assessment of spoken language*. Los Angeles: WPA.

Carrow-Woolfolk, E. (2017). *Comprehensive assessment of spoken language* (2nd ed.). Torrance, CA: WPS.

Coplan, J. (1993). *Early language milestone scale* (2nd ed.). Austin, TX: Pro-Ed.

Dawson, J., Stout, C., Eyer, J., Tattersall, P., Fonkalsrud, J., & Croley, K. (2005). *Structured photographic expressive language test-preschool* (2nd ed.). DeKalb, IL: Janelle.

Dunn, L., & Dunn, D. (2007). *Peabody picture vocabulary test* (4th ed.). San Antonio, TX: Pearson.

Fenson, L., Marchman, V., Thal, D., Dale, P., Reznick, J. S., & Bates, E. (2007). *MacArthur-bates communicative development inventories* (2nd ed.). Baltimore, MD: Brookes.

Fluharty, N. (2001). *Fluharty preschool speech and language screening test* (2nd ed.). Austin, TX: Pro-Ed.

Fudala, J. (2000). *Arizona articulation proficiency scale* (3rd ed.). Los Angeles, CA: WPS.

Frankenburg, W., Dodds, J., Archer, P., Bresnick, B., Maschka, P., Edelman, N., et al. (1992). *Denver developmental screening test-2*. Denver, CO: Denver Developmental Materials.

Gardner, M., & Brownell, R. (2000a). *Expressive one-word picture vocabulary test*. Novato, CA: Academic Therapy Publications.

Gardner, M., & Brownell, R. (2000b). *Receptive one-word picture vocabulary test*. Novato, CA: Academic Therapy Publications.

Glascoe, F. (1998). *Parent's evaluation of developmental status*. Nolensville, TN: Ellsworth & Vandermeer Press.

Goldman, R., & Fristoe, M. (2000). *Goldman-Fristoe test of articulation* (2nd ed.). San Antonio, TX: Pearson.

Hodson, B. (2004). *Hodson assessment of phonological patterns* (3rd ed.). Austin, TX: Pro-Ed.

Hresko, W., Reid, K., & Hammill, D. (1999). *Test of early language development* (3rd ed.). Austin, TX: Pro-Ed.

McCauley, R. (2001). *Assessment of language disorders in children*. Mahwah, NJ: Lawrence Erlbaum.

Newcomer, P., & Hammill, D. (2008). *Test of language development-primary* (4rd ed.). Austin, TX: Pro-Ed.

Prelock, P. A., Hutchins, T. L., & Glascoe, F. (2008). Speech-language disorders: How to identify the most common and least diagnosed disability of childhood. *The Medscape Journal of Medicine*. Available at http://www.ncbi.nlm.nih.gov/pmc/articles/PMC2491683/#!po=1.02041

Prelock, P., Gulbronson, M., Hutchins, T., Green, E., & Glascoe, F. (2013). Psychosocial risk, language development, and bilingual/dual language learners. In F. P. Glascoe, K. P. Marks, J. K. Poon, & M. M. Macias (Eds.), *Identifying & addressing developmental-behavioral problems: A practical guide for medical and non-medical professionals, trainees, researchers and advocates* (pp. 199–234). Nolensville, UN: PEDStest.com, LLC..

Rescorla, L. (1989). The *Language Development Survey*: A screening tool for delayed language in toddlers. *Journal of Speech and Hearing Disorders, 54*, 587–599.

Secord, W., & Donahue, J. (2002). *Clinical assessment of articulation and phonology*. Greenville, SC: Super Duper Publications.

Semel, E., Wiig, W., & Secord, W. (2004). *Clinical evaluation of language Fundamentals-4 screening test*. San Antonio, TX: Pearson.

Semel, E., Wiig, W., & Secord, W. (2013). *Clinical evaluation of language Fundamentals-5*. San Antonio, TX: Pearson.

Squires, J., Potter, L., & Bricker, D. (2014). *Ages and stages questionnaire-3*. Baltimore, MD: Brookes.
Torgessen, J., & Bryant, F. (2004). *Test of phonological awareness*. Austin, TX: Pro-Ed.
Wagner, R., Torgesen, J., Rashotte, C., & Pearson, N. (2013). *Comprehensive test of phonological processing* (2nd ed.). Austin, TX: Pro-Ed.
Williams, K. (2007). *Expressive vocabulary test* (2nd ed.). San Antonio, TX: Pearson.

Resources

Prelock, P. A., Hutchins, T. L., & Glascoe, F. (2008). Speech-language disorders: How to identify the most common and least diagnosed disability of childhood. *The Medscape Journal of Medicine*. Available at http://www.ncbi.nlm.nih.gov/pmc/articles/PMC2491683/#!po=1.02041
http://www.asha.org/public/
http://identifythesigns.org/
http://identifythesigns.org/wp-content/uploads/2013/09/ASHA_Identify-the-Signs_Fact-Sheet-Final.pdf
http://www.asha.org/About/news/Early-Detection-Poll-Results/
http://www.asha.org/NAHSA/
http://www.nectac.org/~pdfs/pubs/outcomesofearlyintervention.pdf

Chapter 4
Principles and Practices Guiding Children's Health and Educational Needs

Introduction

We know that diagnostic and treatment planning processes are extremely stressful for parents. We also know that the care and education plans that are developed to support a child with a neurodevelopmental disability often fail to include full parent participation (Keenan, Dillenburger, Doherty, Byrne, & Gallagher, 2010). This results in ongoing frustration in care and service provision. The role of physicians and other healthcare providers is important in delivering family-centered and culturally competent care. For children and families to benefit from what we know about services and the processes and procedures which dictate those services, we must understand the elements of family-centered care and guide our discussions around those principles. We must also understand the strengths that families bring to a situation and empower families to build on those strengths. This chapter highlights the key elements of patient- and family-centered care and the principles for capitalizing on a "strengths perspective" in practice. In addition, the needed collaboration between family members of children with special needs and healthcare providers is explained. Further, the role of coordinated plans to deliver care is highlighted through a medical home model and other case management approaches to support the health and educational success of children with special needs, many of whom have communication disorders. Finally, strategies to support the educational planning for children with special education needs and strategies for ensuring that service provision is delivered in a culturally competent way are discussed.

Elements of Family-Centered Care

The care of children with special health needs has been guided by eight elements of family-centered care (Shelton & Stepanek, 1994). It is critical that healthcare providers understand those elements and how to incorporate them into their practice.

P. A. Prelock, T. L. Hutchins, *Clinical Guide to Assessment and Treatment of Communication Disorders*, Best Practices in Child and Adolescent Behavioral Health Care, https://doi.org/10.1007/978-3-319-93203-3_4

The first involves the fact that the family is the constant in a child's life, so recognizing their role is critical to a successful health and educational plan for a child with special needs. Second, outcomes are best when a true collaboration exists between the family and other professionals or providers. Third, it is important that information shared with families is complete and unbiased. It is not the role of the provider or professional working with a family to determine what a family should or should not hear or what they might understand. It is instead the role of the provider to share information that is easily understood and provide opportunities for further discussion, often inviting others at the family's request who might be able to support the family. A fourth element of family-centered care is honoring the diversity of the family, recognizing that different cultural beliefs, values, and experiences will influence a family's decision-making and participation in the care or support recommended for their child (Vargas & Prelock, 2004). Fifth, providers must recognize that families will have different coping methods for addressing the needs of their children with special needs which makes it crucial that policies and programs for services are implemented in a supportive and collaborative manner. Sixth, families benefit from connecting with other families who share their experiences, so creating opportunities to facilitate family to family networking is invaluable. A seventh element challenges providers to ensure there are flexible and responsive systems in place to support the intervention and educational practices for children with special needs. Finally, care for children with special needs and their families should always be grounded in their strengths. This strengths-based perspective will be further discussed below.

The Institute for Patient and Family-Centered Care (http://www.ipfcc.org/) established four principles of care for all patients and their families. Although these principles might be seen as most relevant to individuals with medical healthcare needs, all children with neurodevelopmental disabilities and communication disorders have healthcare and educational needs that require attention to ensure their full participation in their community. The first is grounded in dignity and respect such that healthcare providers are to listen to and honor the perspectives and choices of individuals and their families so that the delivery of care incorporates the families' values and beliefs. The second principle is similar to an element described previously and relates to the importance of sharing timely, complete, and accurate information so that individuals and their families can participate effectively in their care and decision-making. Participation is the third principle which asks providers to encourage and support individuals and their families in their care and decision-making. Finally, collaboration is key in the fourth principle which suggests providers, individuals, and families work together to establish policy, develop programs, and implement the delivery of care. Ultimately, patient- and family-centered care requires providers to work "with" patients and their families as partners versus doing things "for" or "to" them. This goal is appropriate for all settings, services, and supports.

The evolution of patient- and family-centered care requires us to reexamine our past approaches to healthcare. Often health and education providers are involved in systems-centered care in which the system drives intervention so that the system's needs and benefits are primary. In healthcare arenas, there is also a focus on patient-focused care where the strengths and needs of the patient are considered but opportunities to partner with the family may be neglected. A more family-focused approach to care sees the family as the unit of intervention but does not consider how the individual functions as part of that family system nor does it consider how one might partner within a larger system of care. In patient- and family-centered care, the priorities and choices of both the individual and the family drive implementation of care (www.ipfcc.org).

Principles for a Strengths Perspective in Practice

The role of a strengths perspective in practice is important because it builds on the principles of family-centered care by recognizing the value of working with the strengths children and their families bring to an intervention or care plan. There are several elements to a strengths-based perspective beginning with an understanding of the potential, hopes, and dreams of a child and the family as well as an acknowledgment of existing challenges (Saleebey, 1996, 1997). A strengths perspective honors the knowledge families bring to education and care planning, recognizes resilience, and creates a context of empowerment (Saleebey, 1996, 1997). Following a strengths perspective in care acknowledges that everyone "belongs" and telling the "family story" helps providers understand who the family is, what they have experienced, and how they have flourished in spite of many challenges.

Kisthardt (1997) outlines six principles of the strengths perspective that providers can consider in their practice. First, whatever help or support is provided, it should build on the strengths that already exist for a family. Second, establishing a relationship with a child and the family is essential to successful implementation of a care plan. Third, families should direct the kind and frequency of the help they feel will be most beneficial for their child and family. Fourth, providers must recognize that everyone has the capacity to learn, grow, and change, so dialogue and intervention planning should recognize these inherent abilities. Fifth, the most effective support occurs in the natural environment where the child and family live and learn. Finally, providers should identify and use the family's natural supports to advance a plan of care for a child with special needs. When providers know the hopes and dreams of families, understand their priorities and need for assistance, consider their cultural values and routines, capitalize on existing resources, and establish collaborative partnerships, they will experience valued outcomes in their work with families (Winton, 1996).

Collaboration Among Parents and Service Providers

To strengthen our efforts in patient- and family-centered care, the Patient Experience Council identified six guiding principles to support collaboration among parents and providers that, if followed, can not only improve quality, safety, and patient satisfaction but also improve the satisfaction of the providers themselves (http://www.ajmc.com/newsroom/New-Guiding-Principles-for-Patient-Centered-Care#sthash.Jzprv1Be.dpuf). These principles have relevance to the work of providers with families who have children with special health needs, including those with communication disorders.

An important early principle of care is the definition of roles. It is important that members of a care or educational team have clearly defined roles that are communicated to the child, family, or whomever is responsible for the child's care. It is also important that members of the care or educational team have the knowledge, skills, and expertise to deliver the needed care and have assessed the ability of the individual child to participate in his or her care and decision-making. Options for intervention or care should reflect the goals, priorities, values, and unique situations of the family and child with full informed consent. Information about a child's care should also be accurate, clear, timely, and easily accessible. Finally, only those who are authorized to deliver an educational or healthcare plan should have access to child and family information. Following these principles for care ensures a collaborative ethic such that team members are sharing responsibility for problems and accountability for resolution. Such collaboration takes time, and engaging families in problem resolution deserves the time it takes.

It is important, though, to recognize the barriers to parent-professional collaboration. Often there is a lack of training in how to work together as equal partners.

There may also be a lack of knowledge and understanding of the ways in which effective listening and speaking can occur (Prelock, 2006). Successful collaboration requires a commitment to family-centered care, recognizes families as the constant presence in the life of a child, helps families prioritize concerns, meets the child and family where they are, articulates the cultural biases of providers which may be different from that of the family's, supports listening to ensure understanding, and solicits family stories to help establish context (Vargas & Prelock, 2004).

Medical Home Model for Children with Special Needs

The American Academy of Pediatrics (AAP) suggests that all children with disabilities have a "medical home" that provides for their ongoing care (AAP, 1992). The original policy statement was adjusted to provide a more comprehensive interpretation and expanded view in response to some of the challenges in early implementation (AAP, 2002). The medical home is an office-based practice committed to partnering with families who have children with special health needs so that care is accessible, comprehensive, coordinated, compassionate, and culturally effective. Some pediatric practices use a care coordinator to help facilitate timely and effective interactions among families, the child's education teams, and other health specialists. As part of the medical home concept, relevant information about a child's medical care plan is exchanged with educational teams to support the child's success in school. Adding care coordination and exchanging information among health and education specialists while partnering with families make a positive difference in the care of children with special health needs and their families in pediatric practices. This approach to care is important for children with neurodevelopmental disabilities including those with communication disorders as they often have difficulties with hearing, vision, behavior, sleep, toileting, and transitions and may have related physical conditions that complicate their function.

A medical home model requires coordination among interdisciplinary personnel (e.g., psychologists, speech-language pathologists, audiologists, occupational therapists), agencies (e.g., schools, developmental and mental health agencies), and health specialists (e.g., psychiatrists, neurologists, and developmental pediatricians) (Prelock, 2006). Care for children with special health needs requires a continuity of services, thoughtful interpretation of shared information, accurate record keeping, and communication among all professionals involved in the child's care. Primary care physicians who support a medical home model for children with disabilities learn a great deal about specific developmental disorders and their health implications.

Coordinated Care for Children with Special Needs

The literature presents a number of case management models for coordinating the care of children with special needs including approaches in early intervention, education, healthcare, and social work (Appleton et al., 1997; Freedman, Pierce, & Reiss, 1987; Gonzalez-Calvo, Jackson, Hansford, Woodman, & Remington, 1997; Jackson, Finkler, & Robinson, 1992; Steele, 1993). Case management is the process typically used to coordinate services for individuals with special needs, although there are diverse interpretations and applications of case management (Etheridge, 1989). A shift in terminology has also evolved from case management to care coordination with the later term more accurately describing the service provision required for children with complex health and developmental needs (Prelock, 2006).

In the healthcare arena, nurses and social workers have been primarily responsible for care coordination with a goal of achieving targeted outcomes in an efficient and effective manner (Etheridge, 1989; Weil & Karls, 1985). Social work as a discipline emphasizes the provision of individualized services and connections to community services and informal support networks (Fiene & Taylor, 1991; Rothman, 1991). Whatever discipline is involved in care coordination, an effective process for identifying needed services and facilitating coordination of those services is critical.

Care coordination within medical homes might include a number of practices. Care conferences are common in the primary care office or at an alternative community site (e.g., school or agency) involving the participation of key members of a child's community team or teams (Prelock, 2006). Key members include not only families but the child as appropriate, health personnel from the child's medical home and school, developmental services providers, educational case managers, and related service providers (e.g., occupational therapist, physical therapist, speech-language pathologist psychologist). Care conference agendas should allow sufficient time for discussion, sharing information, problem solving, action planning, and tracking progress on previously assigned tasks (Prelock, 2006). Minutes should be taken with action plans and those responsible listed to ensure follow-through. Although care conferences require a time commitment, it is likely that the time spent addressing a child's needs in a care conference may be more efficient than managing multiple phone calls and isolated attempts to problem solve.

Strategies to Support the Healthcare of Children with Communication Disorders

Several strategies can improve the health and quality of life for children with communication disorders. Routine healthcare maintenance like hearing and vision screening, use of a preventive medical checklist specific to the child's concomitant conditions, and maintenance of a problem-oriented medical record to address identified concerns (e.g., poor comprehension, unintelligibility, fluctuating hearing loss, learning difficulty, peer problems, inconsistent communication system used across settings, possible seizure activity, inattention) are possible strategies. At a minimum, children with communication disorders should be seen for routine health maintenance visits at the prescribed intervals for children without disabilities. Working closely with parents and related service providers (e.g., speech-language pathologists, audiologists, occupational therapists, and behavioral interventionists) is a must when working with children who might be nonverbal or limited in their verbal communication, have variable receptive language and cognition, have hearing loss, and/or exhibit behavioral difficulties.

Other practitioners who are part of the medical or educational team for a child with a communication disorder have equal responsibility for communicating with primary healthcare providers about the healthcare and educational needs of the child with a communication disorder. For example, establishing a communication system for children with limited communication ability, a speech-language pathologist (SLP) can develop a communication system for answering simple questions, identifying pain, and asking questions. The SLP might also prepare a script or short story describing what is going to happen to prime the child with a communication disorder for a primary care visit. An occupational therapist might share strategies to check the child's blood pressure, take his or her temperature, or examine the child's oral cavity in ways that will lessen the child's oral sensitivity.

Supporting the Educational Plan for Children with Special Needs

The educational plan for children with neurodevelopment disabilities, including those with communication disorders, requires an individualized approach to address the child's special education needs. In the USA, the Individual Family

Service Plan (IFSP), for children birth to two, or the Individual Education Plan (IEP), for children and youth three to 21, is the common pathway to early intervention or service delivery in the schools. Services are generally determined by a child's identified strengths and challenges, a prioritization of goals, and strategies for monitoring progress (Martin & Hauth, 2015). Effective collaborations with families and other healthcare providers ensure service connections at home and school – ultimately improving outcomes for children (Stroggilos & Xanthacou, 2006).

Notably, the Individuals with Disabilities Act of 2004 requires that educational programs implement evidence-based practices for children with special education needs (Zirkel, 2011) including those with a communication disorder when that disorder impacts access to a free and appropriate education and limits the child's ability to learn and fully participate in their educational community. Unfortunately, evidence-based practices are not always available, so careful consideration must be given to an individual child's needs using assessment protocols to document that need (Ryan, Hughes, Katsiyannis, McDaniel & Sprinkle, 2011).

A well-researched curriculum planning structure used to support the needs of all learners is Universal Design for Learning (UDL, Center for Applied Special Technology [CAST], 2011). Educational programs implementing UDL effectively define what a child needs to learn, how they will learn it, and why it is important. A UDL curriculum structure provides choice, differentiation, and alternative learning opportunities for children with disabilities versus just making accommodations for their disability. For example, teachers might present information and engage their students in consideration of their individual learning styles, recognizing each student brings a unique set of strengths and challenges to learning (CAST, 2011). A UDL curricular approach is flexible, customized, and multimodal. It can be used to foster language comprehension and production in children with communication disorders in the educational environment.

Considerations for Culturally Competent Care

Cultural Diversity, Linguistic Variation, and Second-Language Learning Part of providing family-centered care involves consideration of the service provider's cultural competence for working with families and clients from culturally and linguistically diverse communities. Culturally competent care is crucial for ensuring that services are provided in ways that respect the client's ideas and attitudes toward disability, diagnosis, and treatment, for establishing rapport and trust with families, and for ultimately providing services that lead to the best child developmental outcomes.

Throughout this book, the authors have infused a discussion of cultural considerations to highlight the issues that are most likely to arise or may be uniquely pertinent to a particular clinical condition. That said, there are several considerations that transcend the level of the specific clinical condition and are universally applicable to culturally competent care among speech-language pathologists and related professionals. These include the concept of cultural diversity, linguistic variation, and second-language learning and their relevance to assessment and intervention of language disorders in children.

Cultural diversity is commonly referred to as "multiculturalism" which is an umbrella term for regional, ethnic, social, racial, religious, linguistic, and cultural variations within and between societies (Reed, 2012). Linguistic variation is also common not only across but also within countries and takes the form of different languages and different dialects that vary from one another in grammar, vocabulary, and phonology. To complicate matters, most language-speaking communities endorse a "standard" dialect. While so-called standard or "mainstream" dialects are no more valid or correct from a linguistic standpoint (i.e., all variations of a language are both natural and rule-governed), "standard" forms tend to be the more socially accepted and valued form, and tends to be associated with a more educated class (Reed, 2012). As such, it is important that professionals be aware that speakers of a nonstandard dialect are not ignorant of how language works; neither does their nonstandard way of speaking and communicating represent any kind of language or learning disorder. Of course, professionals are sometimes confronted with the question of the potential for a language difference vs. a language disorder. When professionals are uncertain whether they are encountering a language form that is disordered, versus merely different, a good way to begin an investigation involves interviewing caregivers to determine whether they have specific concerns involving their child's speech or language development and whether they think the child's language is typical compared to other children within that linguistic community. Of course, professionals are also encouraged to consult the literature to learn more about a particular cultural or linguistic variation and several excellent sources available for use with American society (e.g., Battle, 2012; Tseng & Streltzer, 2008).

When children are raised in homes or communities where they are exposed to more than one language, it is important to realize that these children can evidence minor delays in their developmental milestones (e.g., first words, first two- and three-word combinations, particular sound combinations) although such delays rarely raise to the level where parents become concerned about their children's language learning. On the other hand, formal assessment of language development in bilingual children can be challenging. The development of bi- or multilingualism in children is complex and depends on many factors (e.g., which language is the child exposed to most?), and it is not uncommon for a child to be more competent in one language than another. This, in turn, has implications for assessment such that children who are learning more than one language will likely evidence variable language skills depending on which language is being tested. When working with very young children who are speaking and communicating and who seem to be on track for their language and social developmental milestones (but who may still be "sorting out" language grammars, vocabularies, and sound systems), one defensible strategy is to take a wait-and-see approach. For young (or older) children whose caregivers are expressing concerns about the child's receptive or expressive language, joint attention, or communicative gestures (e.g., understanding and engaging in pointing, reaching combined with looking), multiple language learning is likely not the culprit, and the child should be referred for a comprehensive speech and language evaluation. Even then, however, it is critical to note that cultural differences have implications for formal assessment including threats posed by testing bias (e.g., using norms based on samples that are very different than the target individual, using tests that contain language that is not culturally or linguistically meaningful) (Reed, 2012).

Developing Cultural Competence As Battle (2012) rightly noted, "understanding another culture is a continuous, not discrete, process" (p. 16). Indeed, the development of cultural competence is also a lifelong process. While we may not develop it fully or apply it expertly in the context of all the diverse populations we might serve, it is important for service providers to understand the potential sources of cultural conflict in the clinical setting and to establish strategies for becoming more informed about these conflicts and how to address them successfully. Most fundamentally, the process of developing cultural competence begins with self-awareness and humility and often requires attitude shifts where professionals recognize what they do not know about the language and cultures of the families and communities they serve and seek culture-specific information and experience in these areas. Being culturally aware challenges us to think more critically about our own assumptions for behavioral norms and to recognize when we are encountering a cultural conflict. When thinking about our own cultural assumptions, it is instructive to also think about several cultural continua that are relevant to all cultures but vary in nature and degree. These continua include, but are not limited to, the following (Tseng & Streltzer, 2008):

Cultural continua	
Interdependence	Individuality
Nurturance of young children	Independence of young children
Time is given	Time is measured
Respect for age, ritual, and tradition	Emphasis on youth, future, and technology
Ownership defined in broad terms	Ownership is individual and specific
Differentiated rights and responsibilities	Equal rights and responsibilities
Harmony	Control

According to ASHA (2016), characteristics of a culturally competent clinician include the ability to:

- Simultaneously appreciate cultural patterns and individual variation.
- Engage in cultural self-scrutiny to assess cultural biases and improve self-awareness.
- Utilize evidence-based practice to include client characteristics, clinician expertise, and empirical evidence in clinical decisions.
- Understand the communication contexts and needs of clients and their families by considering communication disorders within a social context.

The degree to which professionals achieve cultural competence or proficiency in their practice can also be viewed as lying on a continuum from least developed to most developed. ASHA (2016) has described these as follows:

Stage of cultural competence	Hallmark features
Cultural destructiveness	Attitudes, policies, and practices are destructive to cultures and consequently to the individuals within the culture are exhibited
Cultural incapacity	Individuals and agencies do not seek to be culturally destructive, but lack the capacity to help
Cultural blindness	The system and its agencies provide services with the expressed philosophy of being unbiased and function with the belief that color or culture make no difference and that all people are the same
Cultural pre-competence	There is awareness and an attempt to improve some aspect of services to a specific population, and clinicians are aware of perceptions, values, and other elements of their own culture and of cultures different from their own
Cultural competency	A stage of acceptance and respect for difference, continuing self-assessment regarding culture, careful attention to the dynamics of difference, continuous expansion of cultural knowledge and resources, and a variety of adaptations to service models. At this stage, clinicians are able to effectively use their cultural knowledge during interviewing, assessment, and treatment
Cultural proficiency	Agencies hold culture in high esteem and seek to add to the knowledge base of culturally competent practice by conducting research, developing new therapeutic approaches based on culture, and publishing and disseminating the results of demonstration projects. Clinicians champion cultural competence in practice by training others' cultural competence, recruiting personnel from diverse cultures, and conducting research that adds to the knowledge base

Summary

Well-trained healthcare providers who serve children and their families with disabilities have genuine respect for families, share information in a timely and accurate way, collaborate with families as partners in the care of their children with special needs, and invite families to participate in the care planning and decision-making for their child. Healthcare providers are also guided by the perspective that families have inherent strengths, and building on those strengths is likely to lead to more positive outcomes. Coordinating care requires sophistication in teaming, time management, and communication among members of a child's educational and health team – a commitment that is likely to make a marked difference in the delivery of care across settings. Although families face a number of challenges when attempting to provide children with disabilities the best possible educational environment, collaboration among the educational and healthcare team is crucial. Moreover, the educational team and medical professionals involved in the care of a child with special needs must understand the disability and the impact of that disability on a child's full participation in the community. The team must also understand the relevant interventions, the evidence base behind those interventions, and the likely stress families feel when attempting to develop the most meaningful program for the child with special needs (Martin & Hauth, 2015).

References

American Academy of Pediatrics. (1992). The medical home. *Pediatrics, 90*, 774.

American Academy of Pediatrics. (2002). The medical home. *Pediatrics, 110*(1), 184–186.

American Speech, Language, and Hearing Association (ASHA). (2016). Available at: http://www.asha.org/PRPSpecificTopic.aspx?folderid=8589935230&section=Key_Issues.

Appleton, P. L., Boll, V., Everett, J. M., Kelly, A. M., Meredith, K. H., & Payne, T. G. (1997). Beyond child development centres: Care coordination for children with disabilities. *Child: Care, Health and Development, 23*(1), 29–40.

Battle, D. (2012). Cultural diversity: Implications for speech-language pathologists and audiologists. In D. Battle (Ed.), *Communication disorders in a multicultural and global society* (pp. 2–20). St. Louis, MO: Elsevier Mosby.

Center for Applied Special technology [CAST]. (2011). *Universal design for learning guidelines version 2.0*. Wakefield, MA: Author.

Etheridge, M. L. (Ed.). (1989). *Collaborative care: Nursing case management*. Chicago: American Hospital Publishing.

Fiene, J. I., & Taylor, P. A. (1991). Serving rural families of developmentally disabled children: A case management model. *Social Work, 36*(4), 323–327.

Freedman, S. A., Pierce, P. M., & Reiss, J. G. (1987). REACH: A family-centered, community-based case management model for children with special health needs. *Children's Health Care, 16*(2), 114–117.

Gonzalez-Calvo, J., Jackson, J., Hansford, C., Woodman, C., & Remington, N. (1997). Nursing case management and its role in perinatal risk reduction: Development, implementation, and evaluation of a culturally competent model for African-American women. *Public Health Nursing, 14*(4), 190–206.

Jackson, B., Finkler, D., & Robinson, C. (1992). A case management system for infants with chronic illnesses and developmental disabilities. *Children's Health Care, 21*(4), 224–232.

Keenan, M., Dillenburger, K., Doherty, A., Byrne, T., & Gallagher, S. (2010). The experiences of parents during diagnosis and forward planning for children with ASD. *Journal of Applied Research in Intellectual Disabilities, 23*, 390–397.

Kisthardt, W. (1997). The strengths model of case management: Principles and helping functions. In D. Saleebey (Ed.), *The strengths perspective in social work practice* (pp. 97–113). White Plains, NY: Longman.

Martin, C. C., & Hauth, C. (2015). *The survival guide for new special education teachers* (2nd ed.). Arlingon, VA: Council for Exceptional Children.

Prelock, P. A. (2006). *Communication assessment and intervention in Autism Spectrum Disorders*. Austin, TX: Pro-Ed Publishers.

Reed, V. (2012). *An introduction to children with language disorders*. Upper Saddle River, NJ: Pearson.

Rothman, J. (1991). A model of case management: Toward empirically based practice. *Social Work, 36*(6), 520–528.

Ryan, J. S., Hughes, E. M., Katsiyannis, A., McDaniel, M., & Sprinkle, C. (2011). Research-based educational practices for students with autism spectrum disorders. *TEACHING Exceptional Children, 43*(3), 56–64.

Saleebey, D. (1996). The strengths perspective in social work practice: Extensions and cautions. *Social Work, 41*, 296–305.

Saleebey, D. (1997). The strengths approach to practice. In D. Saleebey (Ed.), *The strengths perspective in social work practice* (pp. 49–57). White Plains, NY: Longman.

Shelton, T. L., & Stepanek, J. S. (1994). *Family-centered care for children needing specialized health and developmental services*. Bethesda, MD: Association for the Care of Children's Health.

Steele, S. (1993). Nurse and parent collaborative case management in a rural setting. *Pediatric Nursing, 19*(6), 612–615.

Stroggilos, V., & Xanthacou, Y. (2006). Collaborative IEPS or the education of pupils with profound and multiple learning difficulties. *European Journal of Special Needs Education, 21*, 339–349.

Tseng, W., & Streltzer, J. (2008). *Cultural competence in health care*. New York: Springer.

Vargas, C. M., & Prelock, P. A. (2004). *Caring for children with neurodevelopmental disabilities and their families: An innovative approach to interdisciplinary practice*. Mahwah, NJ: Lawrence Erlbaum.

Weil, M., & Karls, J. M. (1985). Historical origins and recent developments. In M. Weil & J. M. Karls (Eds.), *Case management in human service practice* (pp. 1–28). San Francisco: Josssey-Bass.

Winton, P. J. (1996). Understanding family concerns, priorities & resources. In P. J. McWilliam, P. J. Winton, & E. R. Crais (Eds.), *Practical strategies for family-centered intervention* (pp. 31–53). San Diego, CA: Singular Publishing Group.

Zirkel, P. (2011). Autism litigation under the IDEA: A new meaning of "disproportionality"? *Journal of Special Education Leadership, 24*, 92–103 Retrieved from http://nichcy.org/wp-content/uploads/docs/journals/autismLitigationUnderIDEA.pdf

Chapter 5
Understanding Late Talkers

Introduction

Some children are "late bloomers" when it comes to talking. Around age 2, their language comprehension appears normal, but they may use few words and even fewer word combinations. Between 50% and 75% of these children seem to "outgrow" the delay by the time they are 3, but the remaining 25–50% will demonstrate an expressive language delay (ELD) that can persist for years to come (Shipley & McAfee, 2009). "Because expressive language delay, like a fever, is a symptom found in many conditions, children who are slow to talk are a heterogeneous group" (Rescorla, 2011, p. 141). Some children with ELD will be born with known risk factors and identifiable symptoms of a developmental disorder like Down syndrome or Fragile X. Other children who are slow to talk may have autism where the ELD is accompanied by impaired social communication and a pattern of restricted behaviors and interests. Some may have suffered from diseases such as encephalitis or have a mild or profound undetected hearing loss, while others may have experienced severe language deprivation, abuse, and neglect. Of course, for a large number of children, the cause is never known. Nevertheless, the language deficit persists in ways that gravely threaten educational success and life satisfaction.

Thus, there are some important questions for practitioners to consider:

- How do we define late talking?
- How do we decide which late talkers will catch up and which are at risk for long-term language deficits?
- What are some short- and long-term outcomes for late talkers?
- When do we "wait and watch" and when do we intervene?

These are some of the questions that will be addressed in this chapter although our ability to pinpoint those children who will experience persistent challenges with language is limited primarily because of the large degree of normal variability in child language development.

P. A. Prelock, T. L. Hutchins, *Clinical Guide to Assessment and Treatment of Communication Disorders*, Best Practices in Child and Adolescent Behavioral Health Care, https://doi.org/10.1007/978-3-319-93203-3_5

Late Talking Defined

"Late talking" is characterized by limited early vocabulary and a protracted ELD. For research purposes, late talkers have traditionally been identified on the basis of parent report of child expressive vocabulary and early syntax (Roos & Weismer, 2008). The most frequently used measures are the *Language Development Survey* (LDS; Rescorla, 1989) and the *MacArthur-Bates Communicative Development Inventories* (CDIs, Fenson et al., 2007; also see chapter on Language Screening and Identification Measures, this volume). These two measures have been evaluated positively on their ability to classify toddlers with ELD (Rescorla, 2009; Rescorla, Bernstein-Ratner, Jusczyk, & Jusczyk, 2005; Thal, O'Hanlon, Clemmons, & Fralin, 1991), but an important difference is that the LDS was intended as a screen, whereas the CDIs were designed to provide in-depth parent information about child vocabulary and syntactic development. As a result, the LDS takes less time to complete and is less expensive but yields a less comprehensive assessment of early language skills (Rescorla & Achenbach, 2002).

Over the last few decades, researchers have set varying criteria for the identification of late talkers (Roos & Weismer, 2008). Early criteria were an expressive vocabulary of less than 50 words or no 2-word combinations at age 2 years (Rescorla, 1989). However, results demonstrating that these criteria result in a large number of over referrals (Klee et al., 1998) have led to additional criteria. Klee, Pearce, and Carson (2000) significantly improved accurate classification of late talkers by asking parents if they had any concerns about their children's language development or if their child had had six or more ear infections during the first 2 years of life. According to Klee and colleagues, the child should be referred for further evaluation if he/she is 2 years of age and his/her parents report *any* of the following (Fenson et al., 2007):

1. The child uses fewer than 50 words *and* the parents are concerned about the child's language development.
2. The child uses fewer than 50 words *and* had 6 or more ear infections during the first 2 years of life.
3. The child uses more than 50 words *but* is not yet combining words into phrases, *and* the parents are concerned about the child's language development.
4. The child uses more than 50 words *but* is not yet combining words into phrases *and* had 6 or more ear infections during the first 2 years of life.

Other criteria include scores below the 10th percentile on the CDI at 24 months or below the 15th percentile on the LDS between 18 and 23 months (Rescorla & Achenbach, 2002). Despite differences in the criteria for inclusion, the late talker label is applied to children who demonstrate limited expressive language "in the face of otherwise typical development" (Roos & Weismer, 2008, p. 2). One exception to this involves whether the child also demonstrates a delay in language comprehension (Roos & Weismer, 2008). In research and practice, some professionals use the term "late talker" to include children with ELD and a mild comprehension (i.e., receptive) language impairment, while others reserve the label for children with ELD only (i.e., there is no receptive language impairment).

Predicting Outcomes for Late Talkers

For children with delays in cognition, motor, social, and other areas besides language, referral for assessment, and eventually intervention, is clearly appropriate (Paul & Norbury, 2012). But when it comes to language, it is not clear whether children – even those who meet criteria for status as a late talker – are demonstrating an ELD that is troubling from a clinical perspective. This is because, as mentioned earlier, most children (between 50% and 75%) appear to "outgrow" an ELD with time. It is also true, however, that most children who eventually get a diagnosis of language disorder had a history of late talking – those falling in the one quarter to one half who don't grow out of ELD. Although it continues to be frustratingly difficult to pinpoint who will and will not eventually catch up, several predictors have been identified.

Late talkers who eventually "outgrow" a language delay tend to demonstrate:

- More frequent acts of nonverbal communication (i.e., they tend to use many communicative gestures)
- Higher language comprehension scores on standardized measures
- Higher articulatory accuracy
- Higher complexity of syllable structures (i.e., consonant (C) and vowel (V) combinations – CVC, CCVC, CVCVC, VCVC, CCVCC)
- Larger phonetic or speech sound inventories
- Typical speech error patterns

Late talkers who eventually develop a persisting ELD tend to demonstrate:

- Limited and simplified syllable structures (i.e., V, CV, VC)
- Lower language comprehension scores on standardized measures
- A paucity of communicative gestures
- Limited use of verbs or a preponderance of general, all-purpose verbs (e.g., make, do)
- Limited phonetic inventories
- Few spontaneous imitations
- Poor sentence imitation
- Behavior problems
- Frequent deletion of initial and final consonants (e.g., [ca] for [cat]; [at] for [cat])
- Atypical speech and language error patterns (e.g., vowel errors, failure to acquire early emerging morphological forms like plural -s and present progressive -ing)
- Less symbolic or pretend play

Added to this list of child performance factors are the following demographic risk factors for poor ELD outcomes:

- Male gender
- Family history of speech and language problems
- Premature delivery and low birth weight
- Low socioeconomic status (SES)
- Low maternal education

- A more directive (and less responsive) parenting interaction style
- High parental concern
- Older age at intake

One approach to using risk factor evidence in referral decisions is to rely on the most robust factors. Traditionally, these have been family history of speech and language problems or delay, male gender, premature delivery/low birth weight (Nelson, Nygren, Walker, & Panoscha, 2006; Wankoff, 2011), lack of communicative gestures, and low levels of language comprehension (Ellis & Thal, 2008). It is also known that different children will evidence different risk factors. Therefore, another defensible approach to referral, and ultimately intervention, is considering an accumulation of risk factors (Ellis & Thal, 2008; Weismer, Murray-Branch, & Miller, 1994). With this approach, a greater number of risk factors are taken as evidence for greater general risk. Of course, the number of risk factors alone is not sensitive to more specific expectations for social and language development in light of the child's age. For this reason, some specific red-flag indicators by age for late talkers (birth–8 years) at risk for persistent ELD are offered in Table 5.1 below.

Late Talker Outcomes

As discussed previously, late talking is generally identified by the presence of an ELD in the face of otherwise typical development. The ELD is most often characterized by delays in vocabulary and lack of word combinations, but late talkers tend to be delayed in phonological development as well, and they may (or may not) evidence a delay in language comprehension. Upon closer inspection, however, late talkers often exhibit additional subtle characteristics that distinguish them from typically developing toddlers. For example, in the behavioral domain, late talkers as a group are perceived by parents as having "more conduct problems" and higher activity levels than children with no ELD (Paul, 1991). Differences have also been observed in the amount and quality of play. The symbolic play of late talkers has been shown to be shorter and less sophisticated compared to age-matched peers (Rescorla & Goossens, 1992). Not only might late talkers lack spontaneous initiation of thematic play with others, but they can also have difficulty engaging in their own representational play. Rescorla and Goossens described the late talkers in their sample as "at a loss as to how to proceed to use the toys provided when playing alone" (p. 1298). These early, often subtle, differences reveal more complexity in the profiles of late talkers than is generally expected and may be prognostic of later developmental outcomes.

Late talkers with both comprehension and expressive language delays tend to use fewer communicative gestures and remain delayed compared to children with ELD who have good language comprehension skills (Thal, Tobias, & Morrison, 1991). These and other similar findings point to poor language comprehension and lack of communicative gestures as potential markers for the greatest risk for ELD children. The majority of late talkers with good language comprehension (usually measured

Table 5.1 Red flags in language development from birth to 8 years

Age range	Red-flag indicators
0–3 months	Excessive "tuning out" of surroundings Lack of awareness of sound Undifferentiated crying Problems sucking/swallowing/feeding
3–6 months	Easily overstimulated Lack of awareness of sound Failure to orient to sound Lack of awareness of the environment
6–9 months	Infant does not appear to enjoy social interaction No babbling or babbling with few or no consonant sounds
9–18 months	Same concerns as 6–9 months Does not attempt to spontaneously use or imitate words More interest in objects and less in people Limited persistence in communication; gives up if adult does not respond immediately Lack of communicative gestures (e.g., pointing, reaching and looking) Lack of joint attention (i.e., sharing attention with others)
18–24 months	Same concerns as 9–12 months Less than 50 word vocabulary or does not put 2 words together by 24 months Lack of pretend play Child prefers to play alone
24–36 months	Frequent tantrums if not understood Echoing words the child hears (immediate or delayed) Few or no words or multi-word utterances Does not demand a response from a listener Does not ask questions like "what?" or "why?"
36–48 months	Unable to retell the beginning or end of a short story Relies on direct requests (e.g., "Give me the pen") as opposed to indirect requests (e.g., "Can you give me the pen?) Inappropriate pronoun use (e.g., says "me" for "I") Difficulty understanding spatial terms (i.e., prepositions like in, on, under, behind), temporal terms (e.g., before, after), and quantitative relationships (e.g., more, less) Unable to produce sounds like "v" (in vase), "ch" (in church), or "z" (in zebra)
48–60 months	Same concerns as 36–48 months Difficulty understanding "when?" and "how?" questions Difficulty understanding basic color and kinship terms Poor speech intelligibility
60–72 months	Makes inappropriate judgments in social situations Difficulty describing the events of the day Difficulty telling stories with identified problems and solutions Difficulty retelling stories by describing a beginning, middle, and end Difficulty with rhyming
72–96 months	Fails to understand strategies to hide and detect deceit Difficulty segmenting compound words (e.g., sea…shell) Difficulty learning to read Challenges in listening comprehension skills for conversation, TV shows, movies, or jokes Unable to judge whether an utterance is grammatically correct (e.g., what is wrong with this sentence: There are two book) Does not detect errors in speech and language production

Adapted from Prelock, Gulbronson, Hutchins, Green, and Glascoe (2013)

by receptive vocabulary) tend to move into the average range for vocabulary by age 3 years and for grammar and discourse skills by school age (Ellis & Thal, 2008). However, this is only part of the story.

First, not all late talkers move into the normal range. Although late talkers with poor language comprehension are at higher risk (about 8.6%), it has been estimated that approximately 3.7% of late talkers (ELD only) go on to get a diagnosis of specific language impairment (a language disorder characterized by difficulty in acquiring language, particularly grammar, in the absence of any known etiology) (Thal, Tobais, & Morrison, 1991). Still other children will eventually be diagnosed with a language-learning disability or other language disorder. Indeed, "the language-delayed preschooler of today may well become a future student with learning disabilities" (Bernstein Ratner, 2009, p. 349).

Second, even though many late talkers recover and are indistinguishable from, or even higher-performing compared to, typically developing children, many others go on to demonstrate subclinical weaknesses. Because these children score in the low end of the normal range, however, they are not characterized as language deficient by formal standards (Ellis & Thal, 2008; Rescorla et al., 2005; Roos & Weismer, 2008). These subclinical language weaknesses can occur in basic areas (e.g., vocabulary) but seem most pronounced in the areas of grammar (Ellis Weismer, 2007), reading (comprehension, spelling, written language; Rescorla & Achenbach, 2002), narrative construction (Manhardt & Rescorla, 2002), and working memory (Rescorla et al., 2005). This is particularly concerning not only because these subclinical deficits often persist into adolescence (Rescorla, 2009, 2011) but because these higher-order language skills are foundational to academic achievement.

When Do We "Wait and Watch" and When Do We Intervene?

Warning signs among late talkers for a persistent language problem may be subtle, can present in different developmental, academic, behavioral, and social domains (Wankoff, 2011), likely have different consequences depending on the developmental period in which they occur (Rescorla, 2011), and are known to be different for different children (Weismer et al., 1994). At present, we are unable to accurately predict who will have clinically significant language delay during the early stages of language development because of the significant variability in this period (Ellis & Thal, 2008). For late talkers then, the critical question becomes: When do we "wait and watch" and when do we intervene?

One argument is that the data support surveillance ("wait and see") since most late talkers eventually catch up and perform in the normal range on a variety of language measures. This is consistent with the view that "'late bloomers' appear to represent a phenomenon that is best viewed as part of normal variation within the course of language development" (Weismer et al., 1994, p. 865). The practical implications are important because (1) these children may not qualify for intervention services and (2), when available, early intervention to support language (although known to be effective when necessary) is expensive, and it is prudent to conserve such resources for the children who need them most.

On the other hand, it is clear that a substantial number of late talkers, although they may come to perform in the normal range on some language measures, continue to demonstrate subclinical deficits across many language domains with particular difficulty in the area of literacy, narratives, and grammar. As such, monitoring for clinical-level problems may be inadequate in a world where higher-level language and reading skills are critical to academic achievement. "In a society in which the ability to effectively use language to speak, understand, read and write clearly impacts later educational and vocational success, children who continue to demonstrate relatively weaker language abilities than their peers would certainly be at a disadvantage" (Roos & Weismer, 2008, p. 6). Intervention to support basic and higher-order language skills not only targets language growth and academic success but healthy self-esteem and the formation of successful relationships (Robertson & Weismer, 1999; Wankoff, 2011). As such, we argue that when possible, late talkers should be referred for comprehensive language assessment and that those with clinical *and subclinical* language deficits receive language therapy. One rigorous suggestion for monitoring is that it be routinely conducted to detect not functioning in the normal *range* as is typical but functioning at the average or above average level (i.e., the 50th percentile or above) as a justification to terminate services. Early language intervention of this sort may help minimize later effects on learning even when the more basic ELD is resolved.

Of course, there are situations where such a rigorous approach to intervention is not possible due to lack of available speech-language services. When this is the case, practitioners should consider strategies for prioritizing intervention (Ellis & Thal, 2008). It seems safe to say that children with an ELD that is accompanied by intellectual disability, hearing impairment, chronic middle ear infections, severe behavioral challenges, and social or preverbal communicative deficits should receive high priority for intervention. By definition, these children are not merely late talkers as they are experiencing obvious concomitant challenges and intervention is clearly warranted.

A high priority should also be given to late talkers who present with the most significant risk factors. These are family history of language problems or delay, delay in both comprehension and productive language, and little to no use of communicative gestures. "These factors have been predictive of greater risk for clinically significant language disorders over a number of studies and the information is easy to collect using parent report instruments" (Ellis & Thal, 2008, p. 98). Toddlers with an ELD with other risk factors (e.g., low maternal education, limited phonetic inventories, presence of otitis media) would not cause the same degree of concern although the greater the number of risk factors, the greater the risk for continued delay and eventual clinical intervention (Ellis & Thal, 2008).

Toddlers with an ELD with no other known risk factors would represent a lower level of priority when services are scarce. In all cases of early ELD where services are not available, perhaps "the best approach…is to provide parent training in language facilitation techniques, rather than direct intervention" (Paul & Norbury, 2012). Several studies have demonstrated that parent training to support child language development has had positive effects on children's productive language output (Gilbert, 2008; Peterson, Carta, & Greenwood, 2005).

Because risk factor evidence is central to referral and intervention decisions, one final word on the nature of risk factors is warranted – risk factor evidence is complicated by the fact that the weight of a factor can shift with development. For instance, because expressive language skills in typically developing children improve rapidly between 2 and 3 years, the older a late talker is within this time period, the more the child is falling behind on a steeply accelerating curve (Rescorla, 2009) and the greater the risk for poor outcomes. In another example involving much older children, there is some evidence that low SES is a weak predictor of poor outcomes for very young children with ELD but that low SES becomes a more important predictor (even causal mechanism) of language delay as children get older (Rescorla, 2009). As such, collaboration among health professionals and educators is critical if nonspeech professionals are to be cognizant of the warning signs in language development, as well as the possible social-emotional, behavioral, and academic challenges that may disguise underlying communication deficits (Wankoff, 2011).

References

Bernstein Ratner, N. (2009). Atypical language development. In J. Gleason & N. Bernstein Ratner (Eds.), *The development of language* (7th ed., pp. 315–390). Boston, MA: Pearson.

Ellis, E., & Thal, D. (2008). Early language delay and risk for language impairment. *Perspectives on Language Learning and Education, 15*(3), 89–126.

Ellis Weismer, S. (2007). Typical talkers, late talkers, and children with specific language impairment: A language endowment spectrum? In R. Paul (Ed.), *The influence of developmetnal perspectives on research and practice in communication disorders* (pp. 83–102). Mayway, NJ: Lawrence Erlbaum.

Fenson, L., Marchman, V., Thal, D., Dale, P., Reznick, J. S., & Bates, E. (2007). *MacArthur-bates communicative development inventories* (2nd ed.). Baltimore, MD: Brookes.

Gilbert, K. (2008). Milieu communication training for late talkers. *Perspectives on Language Learning and Education, 15*(3), 112–118.

Klee, T., Carson, D., Gavin, W., Hall, L., Kent, A., & Reece, S. (1998). Concurrent and predictive validity of an early language screening program. *Journal of Speech, Language, and Hearing Research, 41*, 627–641.

Klee, T., Pearce, K., & Carson, D. (2000). Improving the positive predictive value of screening for developmental language disorder. *Journal of Speech, Language, and Hearing Disorders, 43*, 821–833.

Manhardt, J., & Rescorla, L. (2002). Oral narrative skills of late talkers at ages 8 and 9. *Applied PsychoLinguistics, 23*, 1–21.

Nelson, H. D., Nygren, P., Walker, P., & Panoscha, R. (2006). Screening for speech and language delay in preschool children: Systematic evidence review for the US preventive services task force. *Pediatrics, 117*, 297–315.

Paul, R. (1991). Maternal linguistic input to toddlers with slow expressive language delay. *Journal of Speech and Hearing Research, 34*, 982–988.

Paul, R., & Norbury, C. (2012). *Language disorders: From infancy through adolescence* (4th ed.). St. Louis, MO: Elsevier.

Peterson, P., Carta, J., & Greenwood, C. (2005). Teaching enhanced milieu language teaching skills to parents of multiple risk families. *Journal of Early Intervention, 27*, 94–109.

Prelock, P., Gulbronson, M., Hutchins, T., Green, E., & Glascoe, F. (2013). Psychosocial risk, language development, and bilingual/dual language learners. In F. P. Glascoe, K. P. Marks, J. K. Poon, & M. M. Macias (Eds.), *Identifying & Addressing Developmental-Behavioral Problems: A practical guide for medical and non-medical professionals, trainees, researchers and advocates* (pp. 199–234). Nolensville, UN: PEDStest.com, LLC.

Rescorla, L. (1989). The language development survey: A screening tool for delayed language in toddlers. *Journal of Speech and Hearing Disorders, 54*, 587–599.

Rescorla, L. (2009). Age 17 language and reading outcomes in late-talking toddlers. Support for a dimensional perspective on language delay. *Journal of Speech, Language, and Hearing Research, 52*(1), 16–30.

Rescorla, L. (2011). Late talkers: Do good predictors of outcome exist? *Developmental Disabilities Research Reviews, 17*, 141–150.

Rescorla, L., & Achenbach, T. (2002). Use of the language development survey (LDS) in national probability sample of children 18 to 35 months old. *Journal of Speech, Language, and Hearing Research, 45*, 733–743.

Rescorla, L., Bernstein-Ratner, N., Jusczyk, P., & Jusczyk, A. (2005). Concurrent validity of the language development survey: Associated with the MacArthur-bates communicative development inventories-words and sentences. *American Journal of Speech Language Pathology, 14*, 146–153.

Rescorla, L., & Goossens, M. (1992). Symbolic play development in toddlers with expressive specific language impairment (SLIE). *Journal of Speech and Hearing Research, 35*, 1290–1302.

Robertson, S., & Weismer, S. (1999). Effects of treatment on linguistic and social skills in toddlers with delayed language development. *Journal of Speech, Language, and Hearing Research, 42*, 1234–1248.

Roos, E., & Weismer, S. (2008). Language outcomes of late talking toddlers at preschool and beyond. *Perspectives on Language Learning in Education, 15*(3), 119–126.

Shipley, K. G., & McAfee, J. G. (2009). *Assessment in speech-language pathology* (4th ed.). Clifton Park, NY: Delmar Cengage Learning.

Thal, D., O'Hanlon, L., Clemmons, F., & Fralin, L. (1991). Validity of parent report measure of vocabulary and syntax for preschool children with language impairment. *Journal of Speech, Language, and Hearing Research, 42*(2), 482–496.

Thal, D., Tobias, S., & Morrison, D. (1991). Language and gesture in late talkers: A one-year follow-up. *Journal of Speech and Hearing Research, 34*, 604–612.

Wankoff, L. S. (2011). Warning signs in the development of speech, language, and communication: When to refer to a speech-language pathologist. *Journal of Child and Adolescent Psychiatric Nursing, 24*, 175–184.

Weismer, S. E., Murray-Branch, J., & Miller, J. F. (1994). A prospective longitudinal study of language development in late talkers. *Journal of Speech, Language, and Hearing Research, 37*, 852–867.

Resources

Clinical Forum: First years, First Words: SLPs Providing Early Intervention Services. (2011). *Language, Speech, Hearing Services in Schools, 42*.

http://identifythesigns.org/

http://podcast.asha.org/episode-27-early-speech-and-language-development-of-children-transcript/

http://www.asha.org/Practice-Portal/Clinical-Topics/

Chapter 6
Children with Specific Language Impairment

Introduction

Specific language impairment (SLI) has been described as a significant language impairment that has no obvious cause and that cannot be attributed to anatomical, physical, or intellectual problems (Owens, 2010). Although it is a prevalent disorder in childhood, it often goes unrecognized or masquerades as inattention or something worse (Leonard, 2014). Many labels have been used to describe the condition including "aphasia," "dysphagia," "developmental aphasia," "infantile speech," "delayed language," "deviant language," "developmental language impairment," "specific language deficit," "language disorder," "expressive language disorder," "expressive-receptive language disorder," "language-learning disability," "language-learning impairment," and "primary language impairment."

The purpose of this chapter is to describe the nature, possible causes, assessment, and treatment of the condition that we will refer to as "specific language impairment" or SLI. The term is not without its challenges. Even if weaknesses in other areas are "subclinical," impairment is rarely "specific" to the domain of language. On the other hand, SLI is the most widely adopted term at present, it is not mistaken for conditions such as autism or intellectual disability, and it avoids the impression that the weakness in language is minor or temporary (Leonard, 2014).

SLI Described

Diagnostic Criteria According to the *Diagnostic and Statistical Manual of Mental Disorders*, 5th edition (DSM-5; American Psychiatric Association, 2013) (who uses the term "language disorder" to distinguish this condition from "social communication disorder" and "speech disorder"), SLI is characterized by

P. A. Prelock, T. L. Hutchins, *Clinical Guide to Assessment and Treatment of Communication Disorders*, Best Practices in Child and Adolescent Behavioral Health Care, https://doi.org/10.1007/978-3-319-93203-3_6

Table 6.1 Exclusionary factors required for a diagnosis of SLI

Exclusionary factor	Criterion
Nonverbal intelligence	Nonverbal IQ of at least 85 or score that remains above 70 after test error is accounted for
Hearing sensitivity	No indication of hearing impairment; hearing tests are passed at conventional levels
Recurrent otitis media	This factor is unlikely to be a cause of SLI, but to interpret language status, there should not be recent evidence of repeated episodes
Oral structure and function	No structural or functional abnormalities
Interaction with people and objects	No symptoms or impaired reciprocal social interaction or restriction of activities
Neurological function	No evidence of neurological disorder

Adapted from Kadervek (2011) and Leonard (2014)

difficulties in acquiring and using language across modalities (spoken, written, sign language, or other). These difficulties are apparent in early development, due to deficits in language comprehension or production, and include reduced vocabulary (word knowledge and use), limited sentence structure (ability to put words and word endings together to form sentences based on the rules of grammar and morphology), and impairments in discourse (ability to use vocabulary and connect sentences to explain or describe a topic or series of events or have a conversation).

Finally, clinical identification of SLI is contingent on the absence of any known causal factors. In other words, alternative explanations of the language impairment must be ruled out before a diagnosis of SLI is appropriate. The traditional exclusionary factors for SLI are presented in Table 6.1.

Language Profiles As stated above, the DSM characterizes SLI by persistent difficulties in the acquisition and use of language due to deficits in comprehension or production that include vocabulary, limited sentence structure, and discourse. Although these criteria indicate deficits in comprehension *or* production, children with SLI tend to show one of two patterns: good comprehension relative to impaired production or depressed scores in both areas. Note also that the effects of SLI extend beyond the areas (vocabulary, sentence structure, discourse) indicated in the DSM-5. Functioning in these areas will be described first but will be followed by a discussion of additional language deficits characteristic of SLI.

Although SLI is known to affect individuals differently, the modal pattern reveals areas of particular language weaknesses. With regard to *vocabulary*, children with SLI show a slower pattern of vocabulary growth, tend to rely heavily on a small handful of all-purpose nouns (e.g., "thing") and verbs (e.g., "go," "do," "make"), and have special difficulty acquiring verbs more generally. Children with SLI tend to be slower and less accurate in naming tasks, some exhibit word-finding problems or *anomia* (Newman & German, 2002), and the word descriptions of children with SLI often lack detail when compared to those of their typically developing (TD) peers (Mainela-Arnold, Evans, & Coady, 2010). These vocabulary deficits sometimes result in *circumlocution*, a clumsy and roundabout way of talking. Bernstein-Ratner (2013, p. 293) offers the following examples of circumlocutions occurring in the context of naming tasks: "something round and English" (for an English muffin), "on my brother's pants" (zipper), and "you eat breakfast with it" (spoon).

With regard to sentence structure, deficits in *morphology* (putting words together) and *syntax* (putting sentences together) are considered the primary deficits of SLI. As it was with vocabulary, children with SLI are delayed in morphosyntactic development, and although they generally acquire morphosyntactic features in the same developmental sequence as TD children, certain structures prove to be especially problematic. A list of morphosyntactic features that are difficult for English-speaking children with SLI is presented in Table 6.2.

As seen in Table 6.2, many errors appear as errors of omission (e.g., leaving out past tense -ed marking of verbs), whereas others appear as errors of substitution (e.g., swapping "me" for "I"). However, it is important to note that these patterns are not always consistent and can be influenced by other elements (e.g., sentence or word length and complexity, sound production requirements, familiarity of terms) that occur in a sentence (Krantz & Leonard, 2007).

Discourse includes *narrative discourse* (the ability to construct stories) and *conversational discourse* (the ability to negotiate conversations). Successful

Table 6.2 Common morphosyntactic deficits in English-speaking children with SLI

Morphosyntactic feature	Example of error
-ing (present progressive verb)	"Dog eat him food." (The dog is eat<u>ing</u> his food")
-s (plural s)	"She have two book" (She has two book<u>s</u>)
-ed (past tense)	"I walk already" (I walk<u>ed</u> already)
Wh- questions	"What do you think what is in here?" (What do you think is in here?) "What we can make?" (What can we make?)
Prepositions "in" and "on"	"Mommy put table, my book" (Mommy put my book <u>on</u> the table")
Demonstrative (this, that, these, those) without paired noun	"This mine!" (<u>This book</u> is mine)
Pronouns	"Him going" (<u>He</u> is going)
Auxiliary (AKA "helping") verbs (e.g., is, do, can)	"Patty do it" (Patty <u>can</u> do it)
"Be" verbs	"Me Batman today" (I <u>am</u> Batman today) "She baking" (She <u>is</u> baking)
Articles (a, the)	"I want sticker" (I want <u>a</u> sticker)
Possessive 's	"That Mommy coat" (That is Mommy<u>'s</u> coat)
Third-person singular verbs	"Daddy fix cars" (Daddy fix<u>es</u> cars)
Complementizers (to)	"I need go now" (I need <u>to</u> go now)
Three element noun phrases (determiner + adjective + noun)	"The girl here" "The girl big" (The big girl is here)

Adapted from Kadervek (2011) and Owens (2010)

discourse is difficult as it places extreme demands on working memory (e.g., planning and sequencing events) and requires integration of vocabulary and morphosyntactic knowledge, the understanding of conventional story structures and elements, and a sense of audience. The acquisition of discourse skills is extremely delayed in children with SLI. Compared to those of their TD peers, the narratives of children with SLI are less complete, less coherent, and more confusing. With regard to conversation, children with SLI may offer inappropriate responses to a topic and have trouble securing conversational turns and repairing conversational breakdowns (Owens, 2010).

One might expect that children who have trouble acquiring words, constructing words and sentences, telling stories, and negotiating conversations will also have problems in many social situations. It is not surprising then that many children with SLI show marked impairments in *pragmatics* (the social use of language). Pragmatic deficits "seem to directly reflect impairments in language knowledge and use" (Bernstein-Ratner, 2013, p. 295). As a result, children with SLI may act or otherwise seem like younger TD children. Although they use the same pragmatic functions (e.g., requesting, informing) as their TD peers, they tend to express and respond to them less effectively. They may display less sensitivity to a partner's need for information or clarification and be less able to adapt language to suit the needs of the listener. Some children with SLI demonstrate a tendency to interpret language literally, which can have serious social consequences. As Bernstein-Ratner (2013) illustrated: "One child with SLI responded to the subtle indirect request for sharing implied by 'Your snack looks good' by responding 'Yes, and it tastes good too!'. Such a tendency toward literal interpretation will lead a child to ignore the intent behind many conversational gambits… [and] may alienate peers unintentionally" (p. 295).

Finally, *phonology* (mastering sound patterns in a language) is impaired in approximately 40% of children with SLI (Beitchman, Nair, Clegg, Ferguson, & Patel, 1986). As toddlers, children with SLI tend to vocalize less and have less varied and less mature syllable structures (see Chap. 2 for description and examples). Children with SLI often show phonological processes (see Chap. 2) similar to those of younger TD children, but the phonological problems in SLI continue to be problematic in later years and result in reduced speech intelligibility. Not surprisingly, children with SLI also show deficits in *phonological awareness* (how sounds of the language match to letters in the alphabetic reading and writing system) which, when combined with deficits in higher level language skills, leads to *reading and writing problems* and academic failure. Children with SLI can also be very *disfluent* and may repeat sounds and words so often that they are mistakenly labeled as stutterers (Finneran, Leonard, & Miller, 2009; see Chap. 9 for more information about stuttering). One particularly difficult aspect of phonology in SLI is *poor nonword repetition* (e.g., "Repeat after me: flimik"). Challenges in nonword repetition have proven so persistent that some have described it as one of the best diagnostic indicators of SLI (e.g., Owens, 2010; Weismer & Thordardottir, 2002).

Associated Problems Although diagnosis of SLI excludes children with obvious motor or neurological impairment, research has found evidence of *neurological soft* *signs* (Kadervek 2011). Neurological soft signs are not detectable via brain scan but are instead evident in a higher incidence of difficulty with chewing and sucking (Whitehurst & Fischel, 1994). These signs may be interpreted as symptoms of oral-motor weakness or slight motor differences which might be described as "clumsiness" or "accident prone" (Kadervek, 2011).

Depressed *social skills* can be seen in SLI early in development. Compared to TD school-aged children, children with SLI are less successful at initiating play (Liiva & Cleave, 2005) and show more reticence to engage in cooperative play (Hart, Fujiki, Brinton, & Hart 2004). They are also perceived as having poor emotion regulation (Fujiki, Brinton, & Clarke, 2002), are less likely to be selected as preferred classmates (Gertner, Rice, & Hadley 1994), and are three times more likely to be victimized by their TD peers (Conti-Ramsden & Botting, 2004). A practical result is that individuals with SLI experience higher rates of *anxiety and depression*, have markedly *lowered self-esteem* (Jerome, Fujiki, Brinton, & James, 2002), and are at increased risk for social maladjustment into adolescence (Conti-Ramsden & Botting, 2008).

Developmental Course When it comes to productive language, between 25 and 50% of toddlers who are "late bloomers" will go on to have long-term language impairments (see Chap. 6 for a discussion of the predictors and outcomes of late talkers). These children constitute the core of those with SLI (Owens, 2010). SLI in early and middle childhood is characterized by limited vocabulary and impaired narrative performance, but the most obvious signs are the failure to produce simple morphological structures (e.g., omission of past tense -ed or plural -s) and sentence structures (e.g., three element noun phrases like "the big girl"). As children with SLI grow into late childhood, their problems with simple morphology become less severe, while problems with complex sentences, narratives, and figurative language become more obvious (Leonard, 2014). It is at this point that SLI begins to seriously affect school achievement, as deficits in language affect the ability to master reading, writing, and discourse (Bernstein-Ratner, 2013). Thus, persons with SLI are at risk for reading problems, academic failure, and even dyslexia, which is a distinct condition that can co-occur with SLI.

Notably, most children with SLI show gains in language ability over time, but the language deficit proves to be longstanding, and many adults with a history of SLI continue to be less able linguistically compared to their peers (Tomblin, Freese, & Records, 1992). Thus, the language signs of SLI tend to change over the life span, with more obvious problems evident in early development (especially in vocabulary and simple morphology) and more subtle – but consequential – impairments in later years (especially in complex syntax and higher-order language skills related to academic achievement).

Recall that social and emotional well-being is also a concern in SLI. Yet it is encouraging that depression and withdrawal, though detectable, often occur at subclinical levels and symptoms tend to attenuate after adolescence (Leonard, 2014; Records, Tomblin, & Freese, 1992). Although some research has found that adolescents and young adults with SLI may be less independent in daily living (Conti-Ramsden & Durkin, 2008) and may feel less in control of their daily lives (Records et al., 1992), they also tend to hold generally positive attitudes and report levels of personal happiness and life satisfaction no different from their TD peers (Records et al., 1992).

Cultural and Linguistic Considerations

A dialect is a regional or social variety of a language that is distinguished by pronunciation, grammar, or vocabulary. Dialectical and language variation are important to the discussion of SLI for at least two reasons. First, when identifying SLI, professionals must consider whether the child is presenting with a language disorder or a language difference, a distinction that is not always clear. For example, in African American English (AAE), instead of "She *is* baking," it is acceptable to drop the auxiliary verb and say "She baking." "She baking" is an error that would be consistent with SLI in a child speaker of standard English, but a child speaking AAE would be producing language in a way that is consistent with her home dialect, and she should not be wrongly identified as having SLI.

The second reason to consider dialect and language is the striking cross-linguistic differences among children with SLI. As Leonard (2009) explained:

> A common difficulty seen in English-speaking children with SLI is an extraordinary difficulty with tense and agreement morphemes, with omission by far the most common error… In contrast, in languages such as Spanish and Italian, tense and agreement are relatively accurate in the speech of children with SLI, although function words such as articles…can be problematic. (p. 169)

In summary, the morphosyntactic signs of SLI look different across languages. This fact has the potential to complicate assessment (discussed more fully below). One recommendation for meeting this challenge is that professionals consult sources devoted to the description of SLI in the language of interest if they exist (see Leonard (2014) for a review). Another is that professionals consider language profiles at the most general level. "If there is a universal feature of SLI apart from generally show and poor language learning, it is well hidden" (Leonard, 2014, p. 150). Regardless of language then, SLI should be associated with abundant evidence for late emergence of language and protracted development that is suggestive of a delay. Moreover, the errors that are made will *generally* resemble those seen in younger TD children.

Prevalence and Common Concomitant Disorders

Determining the prevalence rate of SLI has been especially difficult due to great variability in how SLI has been defined. At present, the most trustworthy data indicate that the prevalence rate of SLI is 7.4% (8% for boys and 6% for girls; Tomblin, Smith, & Zhang, 1997) making SLI one of the most common disorders of childhood. As noted previously, SLI is strongly associated with reading problems (about 80% of children with SLI experience reading problems; Botting, Simkin, & Conti-Ramsden, 2006) and may co-occur with dyslexia. It also frequently co-occurs with attention deficit hyperactivity disorder (58%; Beitchman, Hood, Rochon, and Peterson 1989) and autism spectrum disorder (3.9% which is about 10 times what would be expected from the general population; Conti-Ramsden, Simkin, & Botting, 2006).

Causes

Some researchers have proposed that SLI represents the low end of the normal distribution of variation in language ability. However, recent research has led to a broader consensus that SLI reflects underlying brain dysfunction at some level, even though it is not grossly manifest (Bernstein-Ratner, 2013). In most cases, there is evidence of a familial, hereditary component to SLI. Of course, this also means that in a minority of cases, the child with SLI comes from families with no evidence of a language disorder. As such, the basis of SLI is complex, likely involves multiple genes and multiple biological factors, and may interact with environmental factors (Bernstein-Ratner, 2013; Leonard, 2009, 2014). Although the quality of the language environment plays a vital role in the treatment of SLI (discussed in more detail below), and environmental contributions to SLI are certainly possible, inadequate language input usually is not considered a causal factor in SLI (see Leonard for a review of the evidence, 2014).

A number of models of SLI have been proposed as explanatory mechanisms (for a comprehensive description of all of the theories and evidence for various models, see Leonard, 2014). Some of the more influential models include the *surface hypothesis* which proposes that children with SLI have difficulty processing those pieces of language that lack prominence due to their sound structure (e.g., unstressed sounds that are brief in duration like plural -s and past tense -ed). Although this hypothesis predicts many of the error patterns seen in the productive language of children with SLI, it cannot explain all patterns, and acoustically enhancing speech to increase the saliency of these forms has not been found to improve performance.

One well-known proposition is the *auditory processing hypothesis.* This hypothesis proposes that children with SLI suffer from deficits in the temporal processing of auditory stimuli (AKA auditory processing disorder where the individual has difficulty identifying, segmenting, sequencing, and integrating auditory stimuli). This hypothesis has led to the development of interventions (commercially available as "Fast ForWord") that have yielded impressive but highly controversial results (Bernstein-Ratner, 2013). In short, a series of studies by Tallal and colleagues (see Agocs, Burns, De Ley, Miller, & Calhoun, 2006; Tallal, 2003, for reviews by authors who have contributed to the Fast ForWord approach) reported large gains on language measures, but other researchers have been unable to replicate these findings. Moreover, the literature on auditory processing in SLI is mixed with some studies indicating weakness in this area (Corriveau, Pasquini, & Goswani, 2007), while others show little evidence of atypical auditory processing (Bishop, Adams, Nation, & Rosen, 2005).

Another model of SLI is known as the *generalized slowing hypothesis.* This model proposes that children with SLI have generally slowed information processing which leads to problems that include, but go beyond, language. This hypothesis suggests that children with SLI need about one third more time to perform a range of perceptual and motor functions (Bernstein-Ratner, 2013). "Such slowing might contribute to, or interact with, other proposals that suggest that SLI is the outcomes of the limited processing capacity in some children. The underlying limit may be one of slowed capacity…or of limits of processing 'space' or vulnerability to competing demands on the system" (Bernstein-Ratner, 2013, p. 299). Additional processing systems that have been implicated include, but are not limited to, deficits in working memory (particularly phonological working memory) and executive function.

Furthermore, Ullman and Pierpoint (2005) have argued that SLI is the result of an impaired procedural processing system, which underlies the learning and performance of skills involving sequences. Much enthusiasm for the *procedural deficit hypothesis* has accrued in recent years as it seems well-suited to explain the heterogeneity seen across persons with SLI. It predicts broad impairment in functions that rely on processing of sequential information (e.g., grammar, rapid naming, working memory, auditory processing) and appears to be consistent with the neurological evidence for SLI (Leonard, 2014). Of course, the actual mechanisms operating in SLI are still a matter of debate. What is clear is that if we can identify the causal factors of SLI, we can develop more appropriate methods for intervention with a focus on early identification.

Assessment

SLI needs to be distinguished from normal variations in language ability. For this reason, the usual recommendation is to avoid a diagnosis of SLI before age 4 years (American Psychiatric Association, 2013). Around this period of development, family members and others close to the child may begin to recognize a language problem although they may lack confidence in their ability to describe it adequately. The child may appear shy, reticent to talk, and prefer to communicate only with family members (American Psychiatric Association, 2013). A positive family history of language disorder (the best-known predictor of SLI) is common, and observation should reveal general language delay with particular weakness in morphosyntax. In fact, the vast majority of English-speaking children with SLI are not identified by their limited vocabularies, poor narrative performance, or possible accompanying speech disorder. Rather, they are identified by their failure to achieve normal syntactic production whether or not they have accompanying deficits in comprehension (Bernstein-Ratner, 2013).

Until recently, low scores on standardized language tests played the primary role in establishing a diagnosis of SLI (see Chap. 3 for a description of several tests that may be appropriate for this purpose). Generally 1.25 standard deviations below the mean (about 80) on a language test would suggest SLI. Some professionals have advocated for a criterion that requires a low score on a test of language comprehension as well as a low score of a test of language production, but this criterion has not been applied consistently (Leonard, 2014). For exclusionary criteria (e.g., nonverbal intelligence), performance in the average range is typically defined as falling above 85.

Of course, the "test score-only" approach should not be considered a comprehensive evaluation regardless of the number of tests. When possible, assessment should also include observation (see Kadervek [2011], for a description of parent-child toy play and book reading observation assessments and assessment tools) and language sample analysis. An added drawback of the "test score-only" approach is that it neglects clinical significance. Indeed, diagnosing SLI using a cut-score of 85 on a test of nonverbal intelligence has not proven helpful because children with scores just above and below the cut-score have been shown to have similar language profiles (Tommerdahl & Drew, 2008).

Recall that diagnostic criteria (American Psychiatric Association, 2013) require evidence that the observed language limitation constitutes a quantifiable *and* functional impairment. As such, some have described the value of test scores combined with clinical judgment and have argued that these factors in combination be considered the gold standard of assessment (Leonard, 2014; Tomblin, Records, & Zhang 1996). More recently, placement into language intervention as an indicator of parent or teacher concern about the child's language development is seen as a gold standard (Leonard, 2014). Another has been curriculum-based assessment where a student's academic performance is evaluated in such a way that reveals functioning across language domains and results in meaningful intervention goals.

Treatment

Productive language deficits are a defining feature of SLI, and, as noted above, whether comprehension deficits should be an inclusion criterion remains a matter of debate. With regard to prognosis, children with comprehension deficits have a poorer prognosis and tend to be more resistant to treatment (American Psychiatric Association, 2013). When gains are achieved, the current evidence suggests modest success when morphosyntax is the target of intervention and success is somewhat greater when treatment targets vocabulary (Leonard, 2009). For treatment of SLI, general language stimulation is not as effective as treatment that focuses on the specific linguistic skills that the child needs to master (Leonard, 2014). Some common intervention techniques that are designed to address the morphosyntactic deficits of SLI are presented in Table 6.3. Of course, in practice, these techniques are often used in ways that can also promote vocabulary knowledge.

Table 6.3 Some approaches to treating the morphosyntactic deficits of SLI

Approach	Description	Example
Conversational recasting	Adult responds to child's spontaneous language by rephrasing it to include the target form	Child: "This green clay" Clinician: "This *is* green clay"
Expansion	The adult responds to the child's spontaneous language by including additional information	Child: "This clay no good" Clinician: "This clay *isn't any* good. It *isn't*. It *is* too dry"
Imitation	Child is asked to repeat model presented by therapist	Clinician: "I *am* rolling the clay. You are too. Say I *am* rolling" Child: "I *am* rolling"
Focused stimulation	Child exposed to large number of exemplars of the target form or work; child may then be asked questions requiring use of that form	Clinician: "Here *is* green clay. Let's make vegetables. Lettuce *is* green. Cabbage *is* green. A cucumber *is* green. Here you make a tomato" (hands child green clay) Child: "No, Tomato *is* red"
Modeling	Adult models a target form; child can be asked to produce form through use of a question prompt	Clinician: "I *am* rolling the clay. I *am* rolling. What are you doing?" Child: "I *am* rolling"
Scaffolding	Adult provides structure for the child's attempts. Gradually, this structure is faded to allow the child to produce the target on his own	Clinician: "This snake *is* very big. This one *is* very small. And this one *is*… Child: "Skinny!" Clinician: "Right. This one *is* skinny. Any this one… Child: "*is* fat"
Sentence combining	Adult gives child two or more simple sentences and asks child to combine them into one longer sentence	Clinician: "The boy is running. The boy wears a red hat. The boy is going to the store" Child: "The boy in the red hat is running to the store"
Sentence expansion	Adult gives core sentence and child asked to elaborate on it and make it longer	Clinician: "The dog is sleeping. Now expand the sentence and tell me why" Child: "The dog is sleeping because he stayed up all night"
Time delay or slowed presentation	Slowing the pace of conversation and waiting for the child to supply a required form	Adult: "All these cans of clay *are* mine!" (pulls the materials toward her and waits) Child: "No, these *are* mine!"

Adapted from Bernstein-Ratner (2013)
In each case, the intervention target is italicized

Most of these strategies were developed from what we know about the kind of caregiver-child interactions that facilitate language growth in TD children, and all of them have received some support in the literature for use with children with SLI. Although conversational recasting has been particularly lauded, it is important to remember that SLI is not a monolithic condition, no SLI intervention is universally effective, and treatment decisions must consider priorities for intervention as well as children's initial ability level and learning style. One common theme from the research, however, is that due to their status as slow language learners, children with SLI require more contact with language targets than their TD peers.

As such, successful morphosyntactic interventions tend to increase the frequency of exposure to language targets while ensuring that they occur in linguistically unambiguous contexts.

It is critical also to remember that although morphosyntax is considered the primary deficit, intervention should not neglect the social and emotional well-being of children with SLI. Social interventions (e.g., peer-mediated treatments) can support social communication and facilitate cooperative play and successful entry into peer groups. Given the potential negative downstream effects of SLI, which include risk for social maladjustment into adolescence and young adulthood, it is imperative that intervention plans address the social dimension.

References

Agocs, M. M., Burns, M. S., De Ley, L. E., Miller, S. L., & Calhoun, B. M. (2006). Fast forword language. In R. J. McCauley & M. E. Fey (Eds.), *Treatment of language disorders in children* (pp. 471–508). Baltimore, MD: Paul H. Brookes.

American Psychiatric Association. (2013). *Diagnostic and statistical manual of mental disorders* (5th ed.). Washington, DC: American Psychiatric Association.

Beitchman, J., Hood, J., Rochon, J., & Peterson, J. (1989). Empirical classification of speech and language impairment in children: Behavioral characteristics. *Journal of the American Academy of Child and Adolescent Psychiatry, 28*, 118–123.

Beitchman, J., Nair, R., Clegg, M., Fergusson, B., & Patel, P. (1986). Prevalence of speech and language disorders in 5-year-old kindergarten children in the Ottawa-Carleton region. *Journal of Speech and Hearing Disorders, 51*, 98–110.

Bernstein-Ratner, N. (2013). Atypical language development. In J. Berko Gleason & N. Bernstein Ratner (Eds.), *The development of language* (8th ed., pp. 266–328). New York: Pearson.

Bishop, D., Adams, C. V., Nation, K., & Rosen, S. (2005). Perception of transient nonspeech stimuli is normal in specific language impairment: Evidence from glide discrimination. *Applied PsychoLinguistics, 26*, 175–194.

Botting, N., Simkin, Z., & Conti-Ramsden, G. (2006). Associated reading skills in children with a history of specific language impairment (SLI). *Reading and Writing, 19*, 77–98.

Conti-Ramsden, G., & Botting, N. (2004). Social difficulties and victimization in children with SLI at 11 year. *Journal of Speech, Language, and Hearing Research, 47*, 145–161.

Conti-Ramsden, G., & Botting, N. (2008). Emotional health in adolescents with and without a history of specific language impairment. *Journal of Child Psychology and Psychiatry, and Allied Disciplines, 49*, 516–525.

Conti-Ramsden, G., & Durkin, K. (2008). Language and independence in adolescents with and without a history of specific language impairment. *Journal of Speech, Language, and Hearing Research, 51*, 70–83.

Conti-Ramsden, G., Simkin, A., & Botting, N. (2006). The prevalence of autistic spectrum disorders in adolescents with a history of specific language impairment (SLI). *Journal of Child Psychology and Psychiatry, 47*(6), 621–628.

Corriveau, K., Pasquini, E., & Goswami, U. (2007). Basic auditory processing skills and specific language impairment: A new look at an old hypothesis. *Journal of Speech, Language, and Hearing Research, 50*, 647–666.

Finneran, D. A., Leonard, L. B., & Miller, C. A. (2009). Speech disruptions in the sentence formulation of school-age children with specific language impairment. *International Journal of Language & Communication Disorders, 44*(3), 271–286.

Fujiki, M., Brinton, B., & Clarke, D. (2002). Emotion regulation in children with specific language impairment. *Language, Speech, and Hearing Services in Schools, 33*, 102–111.

Gertner, J. A., Rice, M., & Hadley, P. (1994). The influence of communicative competence on peer preferences in a preschool classroom. *Journal of Speech and Hearing Research, 37*, 913–923.
Hart, K., Fujiki, M., Brinton, B., & Hart, C. (2004). The relationships between social behavior and severity of language impairment. *First Language, 23*, 343–362.
Jerome, A., Fujiki, M., Brinton, B., & James, S. (2002). Self-esteem in children with specific language impairment. *Journal of Speech, Language, and Hearing Research, 45*, 700–714.
Kadervek, J. N. (2011). *Language disorders in children*. New York: Pearson.
Krantz, L. R., & Leonard, L. (2007). The effect of temporal adverbials on past tense production by children with specific language impairment. *Journal of Speech, Language, and Hearing Research, 50*, 137–148.
Leonard, L. (2009). Some reflections on the study of children with specific language impairment. *Child Language Teaching and Therapy, 25*(2), 169–171.
Leonard, L. (2014). *Children with specific language impairment* (2nd ed.). Cambridge, MA: MIT Press.
Liiva, C. A., & Cleave, P. L. (2005). Roles of initiation and responsiveness in access and participation for children with specific language impairment. *Journal of Speech, Language, and Hearing Research, 48*, 868–883.
Mainela-Arnold, E., Evans, J., & Coady, J. (2010). Explaining lexical-semantic deficits in specific language impairment: The role of phonological similarity, phonological working memory, and lexical competition. *Journal of Speech, Language, and Hearing Research, 53*(6), 1742–1756.
Newman, R. S., & German, D. J. (2002). Effects of lexical factors on lexical access among typical language-learning children and children with word-finding difficulties. *Language and Speech, 45*, 285–316.
Owens, R. (2010). *Language disorders: A functional approach to assessment and intervention* (5th ed.). New York: Pearson.
Records, N., Tomblin, J. B., & Freese, P. (1992). The quality of life of young adults with histories of specific language impairment. *American Journal of Speech-Language Pathology, 1*, 44–53.
Tallal, P. (2003). Language learning disabilities: Integrating research approaches. *Current Directions in Psychological Science, 12*, 206–211.
Tomblin, J. B., Freese, P., & Records, N. (1992). Diagnosing specific language impairment in adults for the purpose of pedigree analysis. *Journal of Speech and Hearing Research, 35*, 832–843.
Tomblin, J. B., Records, N., & Zhang, X. (1996). A system for the diagnosis of specific language impairment in kindergarten children. *Journal of Speech and Hearing Research, 39*(12), 1284–1294.
Tomblin, J. B., Smith, E., & Zhang, X. (1997). Epidemiology of specific language impairment: Prenatal and perinatal risk factors. *Journal of Communication Disorders, 30*, 325–344.
Tommerdahl, J., & Drew, M. (2008). Difficulty in SLI diagnosis: A case study of identical twins. *Clinical Linguistics & Phonetics, 22*(4–5), 275–282.
Ullman, M., & Pierpoint, E. (2005). Specific language impairment is not specific to language: The procedural deficit hypothesis. *Cortex, 41*, 399–433.
Weismer, S. E., & Thordardottir, E. T. (2002). Cognition and language. In P. J. Accardo, B. T. Rogers, & A. J. Capute (Eds.), *Disorders of language development* (pp. 21–37). San Diego, CA: Singular.
Whitehurst, G., & Fischel, J. (1994). Early developmental language delay: What, if anything, should the clinician do about it? *Journal of Child Psychology and Psychiatry, and Allied Disciplines, 35*, 613–648.

Resource

Identify the signs www.identifythesigns.org

Chapter 7
Children with Learning Disabilities or Specific Learning Disorders

Introduction

Children with a learning disability have unique educational needs because of the differences in their approach to learning and their associated social and behavioral challenges. In addition, learning disorders or disabilities often have a language basis and may also be referred to as language-based learning disabilities (Sun & Wallach, 2014). A child with a diagnosis of a learning disability can have a significant impact on the family. There is likely to be an ongoing need to manage the child's difficulties across the life span and to find effective ways to cope with the challenges. Primary care and pediatric practitioners have a critical role in supporting families who have children with learning disabilities. In the paragraphs that follow, a further explanation of learning disabilities or specific learning disorders, as they are currently described in the DSM-5, is provided. A description of the diagnostic process and possible support strategies for this population are also outlined.

What Is a Learning Disability?

Primary care and pediatric providers are likely to see children in their practice who have an identified learning disability affecting the child's ability to listen, speak, read, write, reason, and understand math. The term "learning disability" has been used to describe the discrepancy between an individual's overall capacity to learn and their actual achievement (NRCLD, 2010). Learning disabilities are considered intrinsic to the individual and suggest underlying neurological differences (Prelock, 2013). Although learning disability can co-occur with other disabilities and can be impacted by environmental variables, a causal relationship does not exist.

P. A. Prelock, T. L. Hutchins, *Clinical Guide to Assessment and Treatment of Communication Disorders*, Best Practices in Child and Adolescent Behavioral Health Care, https://doi.org/10.1007/978-3-319-93203-3_7

Table 7.1 Learning disorders as described in the DSM-IV-TR

Learning disorder	Challenge areas
Reading disorder	Letter and word recognition Phonemic awareness or phonological awareness (ability to break up words into sounds) Reading comprehension Reading speed Reading fluency Vocabulary skill
Mathematics disorders	Math concepts (such as quantity, place value, and time) Remembering math facts Organizing numbers to complete math problems
Disorder of written expression	Handwriting Spelling Organization of ideas Composition
Learning disorder – not otherwise specified	Reading, math, and written expression skills interfere with academic achievement even though test performance is not below age, IQ, or education level

The third edition of the DSM-III (American Psychiatric Association, 1980) first addressed the issue of learning problems which were called academic skills disorders. The DSM-IV changed the name to learning disorders in the 1994 edition. The term learning disability was not used in the DSM-IV-TR (American Psychiatric Association, 2000), but the disorders in which it was represented included a reading, writing, or math disorder as outlined in Table 7.1. A diagnosis in any of these areas qualifies a student for educational support because he/she likely will have difficulty in accessing and interpreting information impacting the ability to learn.

The term specific learning disorders is used in the DSM-5 (American Psychiatric Association, 2013) and characterizes challenges in the acquisition and use of one or more areas of academic performance (i.e., oral language, reading, written language, mathematics) persisting for a minimum of 6 months even with intervention. The DSM-5 does broaden the definition in consideration of the latest research. Persistent difficulties in reading writing, arithmetic, and/or mathematical reasoning during formal schooling are required. Common symptoms are slow and effortful or inaccurate approaches to reading, difficulty with reading comprehension, written expression without clarity, problems remembering number facts, or attacking mathematical reasoning tasks (APA, 2013; National Center for Learning Disabilities, 2014). Typically, academic skills will be well below expected scores considering an individual's chronological age when culturally and linguistically appropriate tests of reading, writing, or mathematics are used. Further, an individual's difficulties must not be better explained by other developmental, neurological, vision, hearing, or motor disorders (APA, 2013; NCLD, 2014).

Specific learning disorders are distinct from intellectual disorders because individuals with learning disorders exhibit average or better than average intellectual

Table 7.2 Severity levels for specific learning disorders

Severity levels	Description
Mild	Difficulties in 1–2 academic areas Student performs well with accommodations and supports in school
Moderate	Marked difficulties in one or more academic area(s) Student requires some intensive teaching in affected academic areas and some accommodations to ensure work is accurate and complete
Severe	Significant difficulties in multiple academic areas Student requires ongoing intensive teaching and a range of accommodations to complete work

abilities that facilitate their ability to think and reason. Notably, the current diagnostic criteria do not require comparisons with overall IQ and are consistent with the USA's reauthorized Individuals with Disabilities Education Act (IDEA) regulations (2004) that do not require a discrepancy between intellectual ability and achievement.

The DSM-5 also specifies severity levels for specific learning disorders (APA, 2013). Table 7.2 briefly summarizes considerations for specifying learning disorders.

What Is a Nonverbal Learning Disability?

Although not part of the learning disorders described in the DSM-IV-TR or the DSM-5, nonverbal learning disability (NLD) represents a profile of learning strengths and challenges sometimes seen in children struggling to meet the academic and social demands of an educational environment. Interestingly, a NLD is characterized by deficiencies in nonverbal processing and reasoning, visual-spatial organization, visual discrimination, nonverbal problem-solving, mechanical math, reading comprehension, and social perception (Rourke & Tsatsanis, 1996; Rourke, et al., 2002) with strengths in auditory learning, verbal memory, word decoding, receptive language, and spelling. Children with a NLD often have difficulty establishing and maintaining relations with peers because of their difficulties in social interaction, emotion recognition, and social judgment (Volden, 2004).

Prevalence The Center for Disease Control (2011) reports about 15% or one in seven Americans has some type of learning disability. Considering families with incomes less than 100% of poverty level, non-Hispanic white children (16%) and non-Hispanic black children (13%) are more likely to be diagnosed with a learning disability than Hispanic children (9%) based on data collected between 2007 and 2009 (CDC, 2011; MMWR, 2011). Notably, for children in all three racial/ethnic groups, diagnosis decreases as family income increases. More recent data suggest the prevalence for learning disorders across academic areas that ranges from 5% to 15% for school-age children (APA, 2013) and occurs across cultures and language groups. The National Center for Education Statistics reports the most current percentages for the 2013–2014 school year and identified that more than 13% of public school children (ages 3-21) or 6.5 million are receiving special education services. Of those receiving services, 35% are students with learning disorders. Thus, children with learning disabilities represent a significant portion of those children in special education with reading often being the primary academic challenge (Moats & Lyon, 1993; U.S. Department of Education, 2001, 2015).

Etiology The causes of learning disabilities are unclear although it does appear to run in families and to affect boys and girls to a similar extent. Notably, however, the number of boys versus girls actually receiving special education services is different with boys receiving proportionally more services (Bandian, 1999; Coutinho & Oswald, 2005). Several potential causal factors have been noted in the literature, including problems in pregnancy, birth difficulties or accidents following birth, brain development anomalies, and exposure to toxins.

Clinical Expression It is important for primary care and pediatric practitioners to understand the developmental milestones for toddlers and preschoolers as the inability to achieve those early milestones may be an early sign of a learning disability (Prelock, 2013). Individuals with learning disabilities represent a heterogeneous group with deficits across one or more academic (reading, math, written expression) and linguistic (receptive and expressive language) domains (Fletcher, Lyon, Fuchs, & Barnes, 2007). There are also a number of influences on the clinical expression of a learning disability. For example, neurobiological factors (e.g., genetics) influence the disorder's expression as do environmental factors (e.g., socioeconomic status, educational level, interventions received). In addition, there are core cognitive and behavioral/psychosocial factors (e.g., motivation, anxiety, attention) that impact the expression of the disorder.

Early markers for a learning disability in a preschool child might include speech and language delay, difficulty following directions, a poorly developed vocabulary, difficulty rhyming words and learning numbers and letters, problems with peer relationships, and delayed fine motor development. For early elementary school children, warning signs might include a delay in the child's ability to connect sounds and letters, concept confusion, reading and spelling errors, reversing letters or numbers, difficulty remembering math facts and telling time, and poor coordination (Prelock, 2013). In later elementary school, letter sequence reversals may persist, and difficulty with morphology (e.g., prefixes, suffixes, root words) is common. In addition, handwriting may be impacting written expression, difficulty reading may lead to avoiding reading aloud, poor recall may be affecting comprehension and instruction following, and making friends brings real challenges.

Early intervention can reduce the number of children who qualify as learning disabled (Sternberg & Grigorenko, 1999, 2001). Although classroom accommodations support the student's learning environment, Sternberg and Grigorenko (2001) suggest that schools often fail to recognize the full range of children's strengths and challenges and instructional approaches may not be responsive to children's different learning styles. An integrated approach to identifying and supporting the needs of individuals with learning disability is recommended (Bradley, Danielson, & Hallahan, 2002; Fletcher et al., 2007). This approach considers the value of a response to instruction model for identifying children at risk, evaluating instructional quality, and monitoring progress over time. It also identifies what to do when an inadequate response to instruction occurs. An integrated approach defines a path for more formal assessment in the learning domains as well as a comprehensive evaluation that probes potential language, social, and home factors that could contribute to underachievement (Bradley et al., 2002).

What Is the Process for Diagnosis?

The process of diagnosing a learning disability is challenging as it requires not only accurate testing but also comprehensive data collection through a variety of sources. It involves testing, history taking, and observation by a trained specialist. Several professionals may be involved in the evaluation process including a psychologist or neuropsychologist, an occupational therapist, a speech-language pathologist, and special educator to name a few. During the diagnostic process, a number of professionals may be involved in coordinating efforts to obtain an accurate diagnosis which includes input from teachers, parents, and the student.

Two approaches have been used to identify learning disabilities: the IQ-achievement discrepancy approach and the response to intervention (RTI) approach. In the IQ-achievement discrepancy approach, intelligence and academic achievement testing, classroom performance, and social interaction are assessed. In addition, some students may receive speech-language and attention testing. Assessment results determine if a student's academic performance is commensurate with cognitive ability. If cognitive ability or potential (as measured on an intelligence test) is well above a student's academic performance, then a diagnosis of a learning disability is made. This approach to diagnosis, however, has been criticized because there is little evidence that the measured discrepancy is an indication of a learning disability nor does it predict treatment effectiveness (Aaron, 1995; Barnes, Fletcher & Fuchs, 2007; Harrison & Flanagan, 2005). The discrepancy approach is no longer a requirement to identify a child with a learning disorder in one or more of their academic skills (IDEA, 2004).

In the response to intervention (RTI) approach, the diagnostic process is more treatment oriented. All students are screened early on and those demonstrating some difficulty receive research-based instruction prior to any identification of learning disability. Performance is monitored to determine if providing increasingly intense intervention facilitates the student's progress. Those who respond well to this intensive research-based instruction will not require further intervention or diagnosis, while those who do respond to regular classroom instruction

(Tier 1 support) or intensive instruction (Tier 2 support) are referred to special education and are usually diagnosed with a learning disability. A benefit to this diagnostic approach is that there is no waiting for the student to fail prior to receiving assistance. The 2004 reauthorization of the IDEA permitted states and school districts to use RTI as a method of identifying students with learning disabilities. Notably, this process does not consider individual neuropsychological factors that are often used to design instruction, it takes longer to implement than traditional approaches to assessment, it requires implementation of a strong intervention program, and it is driven by general education versus special education (Fletcher et al., 2007).

In the traditional approach to evaluation and diagnosis, several normed assessment tools are used to evaluate a student's academic performance and achievement. The primary academic domains that are assessed include reading, math, and written expression and achievement tests such as the Woodcock-Johnson IV (WJ-IV), Wechsler Individual Achievement Test (3rd edition) (WIAT-3), Wide Range Achievement Test III (WRAT-3), and Stanford Achievement Test (10th edition) are used. Specialized reading assessment might also include the Gray Diagnostic Reading Tests (2nd edition) (GDRT-2), Stanford Diagnostic Reading Test 4, Comprehensive Test of Phonological Processing (2nd edition) (CTOPP-2), Tests of Oral Reading and Comprehension Skills (TORCS), Test of Reading Comprehension (4th edition) (TORC-4), Test of Word Reading Efficiency (2nd edition) (TOWRE-2), and Test of Silent Contextual Reading Fluency (2nd edition) (TOSCRF-2). Comprehensive assessment is certainly a requirement for intervention as well as helping to determine the contexts in which difficulties are experienced, including the coexistence of language and behavioral challenges.

It is important to recognize that other disorders are often confused with learning disorders and some may co-occur. Typically, those individuals with an intelligence level below 70 on a standardized intelligence test would be characterized as having an intellectual disability (formerly categorized as mental retardation) and would not also be diagnosed with a learning disability although learning will be compromised for this population because of the identified cognitive impairment.

Attention deficit hyperactivity disorder (ADHD) and receptive and expressive language disorders often co-occur with learning disabilities although these disorders are not included in the standard definition of learning disabilities. A child with an attention problem often struggles with learning because of their inability to sufficiently focus on relevant stimuli and organize their responses. A child with a language disorder has difficulties at the core of learning disabilities, affecting listening comprehension and oral and written expression as well as pragmatic language function. All three disorders share executive function challenges (e.g., challenges in working memory, planning, attention shifting) and impact an individual's ability to communicate. These shared clinical manifestations complicate differential diagnosis.

Children with learning disabilities are also likely to have social and language challenges. For example, a NLD has a significant impact on an individual's ability to "read" facial and gestural cues during social interaction (Manoach, Sandson, &Weintraub, 1995; Rourke, 1989; Semrud-Clikeman & Hynd, 1990). This can lead to odd and poor social behavior.

Notably, a majority of the assessed learning disabilities are language-based and children will likely experience difficulty with oral and written expression which is a significant deterrent to their educational growth (Wallach, 2005). Children with language-based learning disabilities may experience difficulty with processing sounds in words, finding the right words to express ideas, comprehending what is spoken or written, understand and using appropriate vocabulary and grammar, sequencing ideas, and organizing and planning their thoughts. The ability to efficiently and successfully communicate often depends on the appropriate use of language in context – if that is compromised, as is often the case for children with language-based learning disabilities, educational achievement will also be compromised. Since language is an important aspect of most academic tasks, students with a learning disability should have a comprehensive language assessment, and any resulting language intervention should be strategically integrated into the classroom environment (Wallach, 2005).

What Treatment Approaches Exist to Support Children with Learning Disabilities?

The National Institutes of Health (NIH) research suggests that 67% of students considered at risk for reading failure achieve average or above average reading performance following intervention in the early grades. As previously described, a conceptual model for intervention (i.e., RTI) is being applied to students with a learning disability so that a school team can determine if a child responds to scientific, research-based instruction as early as possible. A primary focus of RTI is to identify the instructional challenges resulting from the learning disability and then implement high-quality instruction by well-trained educators to differentiate those children with a true disability and those with learning differences.

Treatment for individuals with learning disabilities involves a partnership with all team members including a case manager who implements the assessment process and coordinates the student's program; a special educator with credentials to support the specific educational needs of the student; a neurologist to address concerns about brain function and the implications on learning; a speech-language pathologist who provides support for speech, language, and social communication difficulties; and a psychologist who assesses psychological and intellectual development, guided treatment for behavior difficulties, and mental and emotional health.

Several interventions are described in the literature, and examples are summarized in Table 7.3. To be effective, intervention should be intensive, have a scientific basis, and be individualized to address the specific needs of the student. There should also be a mechanism in place to collect data and monitor progress.

Table 7.3 Descriptions of selected interventions for specific learning disabilities

Examples of interventions	Description
Direct instruction (Hattie, 2009)	Highly structured, individualized, and intensive instruction usually one-on-one occurring on a daily basis; lessons are preplanned to ensure small learning successes and identifying and correcting mistakes immediately; progress monitoring is ongoing
Environmental arrangement or *classroom adjustments*	Modified assignments and testing procedures, preferential seating, quiet space to study and take tests, increased time for assignment or testing completion
Special equipment or *learning materials*	Access to word processors with spell checkers, voice output devices that use text-to-speech and speech-to-print programs, calculators, books on tape, etc.
Classroom supports	Note-takers, readers, proofers, scribes, instructional assistants, or para-educators to support on task behavior and vigilant responsiveness
Special education	Specified hours or placement in a resource room, enrollment in a learning disability program, IEP, and related therapies
Speech-language pathologist	Addresses gaps in learning such as reading comprehension, pragmatics, and written language

See also https://ldaamerica.org/successful-strategies-for-teaching-students with learning disabilities

Implications for Primary Care Providers

For primary care providers, making a referral for a comprehensive learning assessment is a critical first step. A language assessment is also important to determine the level of language impairment that may be involved in a child with a suspected learning disability or learning disorder.

There are also several strategies that can be offered to parents and families to support the language and literacy development of their young children (National Reading Panel, 2000; Stockard, 2008, 2009, 2010), particularly for those families with children at risk or who have a history of learning disabilities. For example, engaging in joint book reading and posing questions about the plot while asking children to predict what is going to happen is an excellent way to facilitate their thinking, comprehension, and story understanding. Retelling and acting out stories is another way to support children's language understanding and use. Family members can increase their child's awareness of print in the environment by having them make grocery lists, read magazines, write thank you notes, read street signs, etc. There are also several electronic applications that can be used to teach letters and their corresponding sounds. For those children with learning disabilities, intervention must be individualized, intensive, and evidence based, and a plan must be in place to monitor progress. Primary care providers are a critical part of the medical and education team that can support families and help to ensure children with learning disabilities realize their full potential.

References

Aaron, P. G. (1995). Differential diagnosis of reading disabilities. *School Psychology Review, 24*(3), 345–360.
American Psychiatric Association. (1980). *Diagnostic and statistical manual* (3rd ed.). Washington, DC: APA Press.
American Psychiatric Association (2000). *Diagnostic and statistical manual* (4th ed., Text Rev.). Washington, DC: APA Press.
American Psychiatric Association (2013). *Diagnostic and statistical manual* (5th ed., Text Rev.). Washington, DC: APA Press.
Bandian, N. A. (1999). Reading disability defined as a discrepancy between listening and reading comprehension: A longitudinal study of stability, gender differences, and prevalence. *Journal of Learning Disabilities, 32*(2), 138–148.
Barnes, M. A., Fletcher, J., & Fuchs, L. (2007). *Learning disabilities: From identification to intervention.* New York: The Guilford Press.
Bradley, R., Danielson, L., & Hallahan, D. P. (2002). *Identification of learning disabilities: Research to practice.* Mahwah, NJ: Erlbaum.
Center for Disease Control (2011). National Health Interview Survey 2007-2009 data. Available at http://www.cdc.gov/nchs/nhis.htm.
Coutinho, M. J., & Oswald, D. P. (2005). State variation in gender disproportionally in special education: Finding and recommendations. *Remedial and Special Education, 26*(1), 7–15.
Fletcher, J. M., Lyon, G. R., Fuchs, L. S., & Barnes, M. A. (2007). Classification, definition and identification of learning disabilities. In *Learning disabilities: From identification to intervention* (pp. 25–63). NewYork: The Guilford Press.
Harrison, P. L., & Flanagan, D. P. (2005). *Contemporary intellectual assessment: Theories, tests, and issues.* New York: Guilford Press.
Hattie, J. (2009). *Visible learning: A synthesis of over 800 meta-analyses relating to achievement.* London/New York: Routledge.
Individuals with Disabilities Education Improvement Act of 2004. Pub L No. 108–446, §§ 1400 et seq.
Manoach, D., Sandson, T., & Weintraub, S. (1995). The developmental social-emotional processing disorders is associated with right hemisphere abnormalities. *Neuropsychiatry, Neurophysiology, Behavioral Neurology, 8*, 99–105.
Moats, L. C., & Lyon, G. R. (1993). Learning disabilities in the United States. Advocacy, sciences, and the future of the field. *Journal of Learning Disabilities, 26*, 282–294.
Morbidity and Mortality Weekly Report. (2011). QuickStats: Percentage of children aged 5-17 years ever receiving a diagnosis of learning disability,* by Race/Ethnicity† and Family Income Group§ — National Health Interview Survey,¶ United States, 2007-2009. *MMWR, 60*(25), 853. http://www.cdc.gov/nchs/nhis.htm
National Center for Learning Disabilities (2014). *The state of learning disabilities* (3rd ed.). New York: Author.
National Reading Panel (2000). Teaching children to read: An evidence-based assessment of the scientific research literature on reading and its implications for reading instruction. Retrieved from http://1.usa.gov/sOnDsl
National Research Center on Learning Disabilities (NRCLD) (2010). *The Learning Disabilities Resource Kit: Specific Learning Disabilities Determination Procedures and Responsiveness to Intervention*, NRCLD (National Research Center on Learning Disabilities). (Available online at http://www.nrcld.org/resource_kit/)
Prelock, P. A. (2013). What is a learning disability? In F. R. Volkmar (Ed.), *Encyclopedia for autism spectrum disorders* (1st ed.). New York: Springer.

Rourke, B. P. (1989). *Nonverbal learning disabilities: The syndrome and the model*. NewYork: The Guilford Press.

Rourke, B. P., Ahmad, S., Collins, D., Hayman-Abello, B., Sayman-Abello, S., & Warriner, E. (2002). Child clinical/pediatric neuropsychology: Some recent advances. *Annual Reviews of Psychology, 53*, 309–339.

Rourke, B. P., & Tsatsanis, K. D. (1996). Syndrome of nonverbal learning disabilities: Psycholinguistic assets and deficits. *Topics in Language Disorders, 16*, 30–44.

Semrud-Clikeman, M., & Hynd, G. (1990). Right hemispheric dysfunction in nonverbal learning disabilities: Social, academic, and adaptive functioning in adults and children. *Psychological Bulletin, 107*, 196–209.

Sternberg, R. J., & Grigorenko, E. L. (1999). *Our labeled children: What every parent and teacher needs to know about learning disabilities*. Reading, MA: Perseus Publishing Group.

Sternberg, R. J., & Grigorenko, E. L. (2001, December). Learning disabilities, schooling, and society. *Phi Delta Kappa, 83*, 335–338.

Stockard, J. (2008). *Reading achievement in a direct instruction school and a 'Three Tier' Curriculum School* (NIFDI Technical Report 2008. 5).

Stockard, J. (2009). *Promoting early literacy of preschool children: A study of the effectiveness of Funnix beginning reading* (NIFDI Technical Report 2009, 1).

Stockard, J. (2010). Promoting early literacy of preschool children: A study of the effectiveness of Funnix beginning reading. *Journal of Direct Instruction, 10*, 29–48.

Sun, L., & Wallach, G. P. (2014). Language disorders are learning disabilities. Challenges on the divergent and diverse paths to language learning disability. *Topics in Language Disorders, 34*(1), 25–38.

U. S. Department of Education. (2001). *Twenty-third annual report to congress on the implementation of the individuals with disabilities education act*. Washington, DC: Author.

U.S. Department of Education, Office of Special Education Programs, Individuals with Disabilities Education Act (IDEA) database, retrieved September 25, 2015., from http://www2.ed.gov/programs/osepidea/618-data/state-level-data-files/index.html#bcc; and National Center for Education Statistics, Common Core of Data (CCD), "State Nonfiscal Survey of Public Elementary/Secondary Education," 2013–14. See *Digest of Education Statistics 2015*, table 204.30 and table 204.50.

Volden, J. (2004). Nonverbal learning disability: A tutorial for speech-language pathologists. *American Journal of Speech-Language Pathology, 13*, 128–141.

Wallach, G. P. (2005). A conceptual framework in language learning disabilities: School-age language disorders. *Topics in Language Disorders, 25*(4), 292–301.

Chapter 8
Children with Speech Disorders

Introduction

As introduced in the first chapter, approximately 8% of children between the ages of 3 and 17 will experience a problem with their speech (Black, Vahratian, & Hoffman, 2015). "Speech" refers to the act of communicating orally by using air propelled from the lungs through the larynx and shaped by movements of the articulators within the pharynx and the oral cavity to produce sequences of consonant and vowel sounds. There are three types of speech disorders primary care providers are likely to see: (1) speech sound disorders, which result in the misproduction of speech sounds and word shapes; (2) fluency disorders, which interrupt the smooth flow of speech; and (3) voice disorders, which impact the quality of the sound stream from the larynx. Each of these is described in greater detail below.

Speech Sound Disorders

From birth or even before, infants' sensory, motor, articulatory, social, and cognitive experiences gradually build the foundation for successful, adult-like oral communication. Almost all young children make mistakes when they are learning to say new words; it is typical for certain types of speech errors to persist for some time. Typical speech development is reviewed in Chap. 2. A *speech delay* occurs when a child makes errors that are more typical of a younger child. A *speech sound disorder* (previously referred to as an articulation disorder) occurs when a child makes pronunciation errors that are not typical at any age or when a child's errors are not consistently typical of a certain age (i.e., chronological mismatch: some speech production skills are more immature than others). A *speech difference* occurs when a child is exposed to a language or dialect or a set of languages or dialects that are

P. A. Prelock, T. L. Hutchins, *Clinical Guide to Assessment and Treatment of Communication Disorders*, Best Practices in Child and Adolescent Behavioral Health Care, https://doi.org/10.1007/978-3-319-93203-3_8

not the same as the languages or dialects of the surrounding community. A speech difference is neither a delay nor a disorder, but it can be confused with these. Also, it is important to note that a speech difference can co-occur with a speech delay or disorder; the fact that a child has a different accent due to the language spoken at home may or may not mean that the child has a speech sound disorder. Similarly, other disorders that impact communication – such as language disorders, autism, attention deficit disorders, and learning disabilities – often co-occur with speech sound disorders.

Speech sound disorders occur for a variety of reasons. Some are the result of structural anomalies such as cleft palate, other craniofacial differences, or atypical muscle tone due to neurodevelopmental syndromes, which can make speech sounds physically difficult to produce. Sometimes speech sound disorders are perceptually based, as is the case with hearing loss or auditory processing disorders. The child could also be experiencing problems with motor planning for speech. Other times a speech sound disorder reflects a linguistic problem, i.e., the child has trouble learning the rules that govern the use of speech sounds and word shapes. Oftentimes, speech sound disorders result from a combination of these factors. Regardless of the cause, human beings often judge each other based on the clarity and precision of their speech. Those with speech sound disorders are often seen as being less capable or less intelligent; as a result, they tend to have the benefit of fewer educational and occupational opportunities (Lewis & Freebairn, 1992).

In this section, we consider physical/physiological, sensory, motor planning, and cognitive/linguistic sources of speech sound disorders. Table 8.1 summarizes some of these etiologies and symptoms, with some key treatment strategies for each.

Physical/Physiological Conditions

Birth Defects Impacting the Palate Palatal clefts, submucous clefts, or other causes of velopharyngeal insufficiency result in hypernasality due to leakage of air through the nasal cavity, which may lead to other difficulties with speech production. The most common, yet often undiagnosed, cause of hypernasality is velocardial facial syndrome (VCF), which results from a chromosomal deletion at 22q.11. Children with a variety of other genetic syndromes (e.g., Prader-Willi, de Lange, Laurence-Moon-Biedl, Sotos, and Noonan syndromes) have high-arched palates and accompanying speech deficits.

Other Craniofacial Anomalies A variety of other craniofacial differences are also associated with speech production challenges, often in addition to velopharyngeal insufficiency. These are due to various syndromes such as fetal alcohol syndrome, craniofacial microsomia, Treacher Collins syndrome, and Pierre Robin sequence.

Other Syndromes or Conditions There are several other syndromes or conditions healthcare providers might see that impact speech production. For example, children with *Moebius syndrome*, which has no known consistent genetic basis, demonstrate

Table 8.1 Causes, symptoms, and treatment strategies for speech sound disorders

Condition	Prevalence (live births)	Primary speech symptoms	Primary treatment strategies
Clefts (lip, palate)	1.5–2.5 cases per 1000	Hypernasality	Surgery followed by speech therapy to (re)learn speech patterns with repaired structures
Cerebral palsy (spastic, athetoid [dyskinetic], ataxic, mixed)	1.5–4 per 1000	Distortions, slow rate, hypernasality	Speech therapy focusing on compensatory strategies; nonspeech exercises do not help
Down syndrome	1 per 1000	Distortions, slow rate, atypical error patterns	Speech therapy focusing on compensatory strategies; nonspeech exercises do not help
Moebius syndrome	2 per 100,000	Limited ability to articulate speech sounds, especially labials (b, p, m)	Speech therapy focusing on compensatory strategies; nonspeech exercises do not help
Ankyloglossia	4–10 per 100	Inability to produce tongue-tip consonants (t, d, n, l, s)	Clipping of the lingual frenulum *in severe cases only*
Childhood apraxia of speech	1–2 per 1000	Choppy, effortful speech with vowel and stress errors; language and literacy deficits	Speech therapy focusing on motor speech planning

complete or partial unilateral or bilateral paralysis of the facial nerve and often also palsy of the ocular (VI), trigeminal (V), vagus (X), or glossopharyngeal (IX) nerves; paralysis of nerve XII results in hypoplasia of the tongue. Oral-facial anomalies are also typical. Not surprisingly, atypical speech production patterns and poor intelligibility result.

Tongue-tie (*Ankyloglossia*), in which a short lingual frenulum ("tongue-tie") has been identified, may or may not have an impact on speech production. There are many long-standing myths about tongue-tie. Now we know that only the most restricted lingual frenula result in speech impairments. Notably, the distance between the upper and lower teeth when the child opens his mouth as far as possible with the tongue tip on the upper teeth is more prognostic of speech deficits than the extent of tongue protrusion. If the frenulum is clipped in order to release the tongue, it is very important for the child to do tongue exercises following the surgery to prevent scarring that can impact tongue movement (Messner & Lalakea, 2002).

Although children with *Down syndrome* (DS) appear to have large tongues, they actually have short hard palates, unusually small oral cavities, low lingual muscle tone, and atypical facial musculature, all of which can impact the accuracy of their speech production (Crelin, 1987). In fact, for children with DS, one large muscle mass replaces many of the individual muscles in the typical face, resulting in limited facial and labial flexibility (Miller & Leddy, 1998). The speech of children with DS is also typically affected by oral-motor problems, hearing loss, linguistic-cognitive deficits, sequential processing difficulties, and motor speech deficits, including dysarthria resulting from low muscle tone and sometimes symptoms of childhood apraxia of speech (see below) (Swift & Rosin, 1990; Rupela & Manjula, 2007).

Different types of *cerebral palsy* result in different speech motor control challenges. For instance, athetoid cerebral palsy (which is typically caused by bilirubin abnormalities or anoxia) is characterized by unbalanced, fluctuating muscle tone, persistent reflexes, spasms, and jerky, extreme movements. Children with this type of cerebral palsy have very poor control of their articulators, and their speech tends to be imprecise, variable, and slow, with inappropriate nasality. The most common type is spastic cerebral palsy, which is associated with decreased motor control and therefore distorted speech, as well as with decreased cognitive ability.

Childhood Dysarthria

Cerebral palsy is the most common cause of childhood dysarthria, the symptoms of which include deficits in respiration, phonation, articulation, resonance, and/or prosody as a result of neuromotor damage or difference, often in the prenatal/neonatal period. Dysarthrias typically result in articulatory imprecision (distortions) and omissions of speech sounds, often due to abnormalities in the motor neurons supplying information to the tongue. Several types of dysarthria also cause prosody and resonance disorders, especially impacting stress and nasality. Slow or irregular speech rate may result in part from inadequate respiratory capacity.

Several other neurodevelopmental syndromes (such as Williams syndrome, achondroplasia, familial dysautonomia, Marfan syndrome, Prader-Willi syndrome, Tay-Sachs disease, Werdnig-Hoffmann disease, muscular dystrophy, Duchenne muscular dystrophy, and spinal muscular atrophy) as well as perinatal trauma (e.g., perinatal stroke) and sometimes autism spectrum disorders (at early ages) may also result in tone abnormalities and therefore in childhood dysarthria. Many are also associated with other syndrome-specific speech production or speech sound learning deficits.

Sensory Conditions

Vision, hearing, and higher-order auditory processes, such as speech perception (the linguistic interpretation of speech sounds and structures), have known impacts on the child's development of spoken language. The impact of hearing loss/deafness on speech and language development is discussed in a later chapter.

Perhaps more surprisingly, infants as young as 4 months of age use their vision to supplement their hearing during vocal turn-taking. Visual factors can have a significant impact on speech perception even in typical adults. However, the impact of blindness on speech development has yet to be thoroughly studied.

Childhood Apraxia of Speech

Childhood apraxia of speech (CAS) is an impairment of speech motor planning. That is, the musculature is intact, and the child knows what word(s) he wants to say, but, as in adult-onset apraxia of speech (AOS), the ability to make a motor plan to carry out the articulation of the word(s) and the ability to generalize motor plans to more flexible motor programs are both impaired. Symptoms typically include effortful speech (sometimes characterized by articulatory groping), slowed rate, choppy rhythm, vowel errors, sequencing difficulties, and inappropriate stress patterns. CAS or CAS-like symptoms are associated with certain genetic syndromes such as FOXP2 (chromosomal translocation in the region 7q31), 7q11.23 duplication syndrome, galactosemia, fragile X syndrome, Rett syndrome, and VCF (22q.11 deletion syndrome). It is also seen in some children with perinatal strokes or other neurological impairments or differences. Most often, however, the etiology is unknown. CAS is also frequently associated with language and literacy deficits. Although at one time a commonly listed primary symptom of CAS was "lack of progress in speech therapy," more recently specific speech-language intervention strategies have shown significant results.

Cognitive and Linguistic Factors

Successful oral communication requires far more than the ability to form sounds with the articulators. Sometimes using a different sound changes the meaning of a word (e.g., substituting the "t" in "coat" with a "d" sound results in a different word – "code"). In other cases, sound substitutions simply reflect stylistic choices (e.g., substituting a glottal stop [the sound in the middle of the word "uh-oh"] at the end of the word "coat" results in a more casual production of the word; the meaning does not change). The sets of sounds that change meanings, called *phonemes*, differ from one language to another. These phonological contrasts are crucial for successful oral expression of a variety of ideas.

Furthermore, a variety of complex rules determine how the phonemes in a given language can be combined to form syllables and how syllables combine to form words and phrases. For example, in languages such as English, German, and Russian, syllables can begin or end with sequences of consonants (known as consonant clusters or blends). In other languages, such as Japanese and Hawaiian, each consonant must have a vowel before or after it. The context in which a phoneme or a morpheme (a grammatical unit) occurs often changes its pronunciation. In English, for example, the past tense morpheme "ed" is pronounced as "t" in certain contexts, as "d" in other contexts, and as "ed" in still other contexts. In French, consonants that occur at the end of a word, such as the "x" at the end of "beaux" (the plural form of the word "beautiful"), are sometimes pronounced (as in "beaux arts" ["boze ar"] – "fine arts") and sometimes not (e.g., "Ils sont beaux" ["eel soh boe"] – "They are handsome").

Children must learn all of these complex phonological rules based solely on their exposure to the language(s) spoken in their environments ("implicit learning"). Some children are good at this and others are not. Children who are learning more than one language must learn multiple sets of rules. This may result in slightly slower phonological development initially, but in the long run, it yields higher levels of linguistic flexibility and understanding.

Children with cognitive-linguistic speech sound disorders may be able to articulate the sounds and structures of the language but lack understanding of the rules that govern those sounds and structures. For this reason, they may overuse or misuse certain sounds, syllables, or words. They need to be explicitly taught the phonological contrasts and rules of the ambient language(s).

Phonological Error Patterns

Regardless of the cause, children with speech sound disorders often exhibit error patterns (often called phonological processes). The phonological processes that are common in typically developing children learning English are reviewed in Chap. 2. The processes of children with speech sound disorders vary based on the disorder. Those with dysarthria, for example, consistently produce imprecise, distorted consonants, such as lisped [s]. Due to their weak muscle tone, they also tend to demonstrate frication, an atypical error pattern in which stops (abrupt consonant sounds resulting from complete closure then release within the oral cavity, such as /p, t, k, b, d, g/) are substituted with fricatives (consonants with hissing sounds resulting from squeezing air in the oral cavity, such as [f, s, v, z] as well as "sh" and "th").

Children with CAS tend to use more phonotactic (structural) processes than children with other speech sound disorders; this can result in omission, insertion, and/or mis-sequencing error patterns within words (e.g., attempting to say "clap" but producing "cap," "clasp," or "plack" instead). They also demonstrate vowel error patterns, which are rare in children who are typically developing. Children with cognitive-linguistic speech sound disorders often fail to learn the rules of their language, to mis-learn them, or to over-apply them. For example, an English-learning child with a speech sound disorder might not understand that /p/ and /b/ are different phonemes and might therefore use [b] exclusively at the beginnings of words (saying "buppy" for "puppy"), i.e., use the phonological process called "voicing," and [p] at the end of the word (saying "mob" for "mop"), i.e., use the phonological process called "devoicing."

In short, the fact that a pattern (or process) can be detected does not indicate the nature of the speech sound disorder. The specific type of pattern that is occurring is much more informative.

Referring for Speech Sound Assessments

Regardless of the languages that they are learning, by the age of 2, a toddler should be using at least five to nine different consonants to differentiate words. They should also be using at least several different vowels appropriately. New sounds should be added, in new word positions and structures (as allowed by the language[s] the child is exposed to), on a regular basis thereafter. Physicians and other primary healthcare providers can identify children who should be referred for a speech evaluation by asking about the sounds that the child is using, how well they understand the words the children say (see "Intelligibility" in Chapter 2), the effort required for the child to produce those words, the rate of progress observed, and whether or not either the child or the parents are frustrated about the child's communication ability. Some expectations for speech sound development are listed, by age, in Table 8.2.

Table 8.2 Expectations for typical speech sound development, by age

Age	Expectations
Any age	Understood about as well as peers Not teased about speech by peers Not excessively frustrated about speaking; not unusually reluctant to speak Not using compensatory strategies – gesturing, acting out – instead of speaking
24 months	More than 5 different consonants[a] and 5 different vowels[a] used functionally to differentiate words in a consistent, recognizable manner Understood at least 50% of the time
36 months	Variety of word shapes used contrastively (to differentiate word meanings): Different numbers of syllables per word Consonants in initial and final[a] position Some consonant clusters[a] – not always accurate Substitutes some consonants for others but doesn't substitute one consonant for many others (e.g., [d] used instead of most other consonant sounds) Vowels are accurate except hardest diphthongs (such as "air," "our," etc. in English) Produces some "hard sounds," although not always accurately, such as: Fricatives (such as [f, v, s, z], and "sh") Liquids or trills ([l], "r") Understood at least 75% of the time
48 months	Uses all word shapes in the language although not always accurately (e.g., uses clusters[a] but may substitute for difficult sounds within the clusters such as saying "gween" for "green") Substitutes only for 2–4 of the most difficult sounds in the language (e.g., for English: substitutes for no more than 4 of /r/, /s/, /z/, /k/, /g/, "th," "j," "ch"); usually produces the other difficult sounds correctly Understood 100% of the time

[a]If included in the language[s] being learned

Treatment of Speech Sound Disorders

Not surprisingly, intervention depends upon the nature of the speech sound disorder. If the child is unable to produce certain sounds or structures for physical/physiological reasons, therapy will focus initially on improving articulatory accuracy. However, *neither nonspeech strengthening exercises (oral-motor exercises) nor practicing sounds in isolation is effective*. Even for dysarthria, for which speech-based intervention focusing on compensatory strategies may result in improved intelligibility and/or vocal clarity and quality for children, nonspeech exercises (blowing, tongue clicking, and other strengthening or stretching activities) appear to have no positive effects on speech (Pennington, Parker, Kelly, & Miller, 2016). Speech requires different types of coordination and rhythm than nonspeech articulatory activities do. Furthermore, producing sounds within words requires coarticulation (coordination from one sound to the next); practicing individual sounds out of context fails to teach these interactive patterns. Therefore, to improve functional speech production, you have to practice functional speech production directly (Forrest, 2002).

Another focus of therapy for children with physical/physiological challenges – as well as other children with severe-to-profound disorders – is intelligibility. It is quite possible to increase intelligibility even if speech accuracy per se cannot be improved. Pausing in the appropriate locations within a sentence (e.g., between clauses), stressing the key words, and using redundancy (e.g., saying "yesterday" as well as using the past tense of the verb) can all make a speaker far easier to understand.

For children with motor speech planning disorders, training articulatory flexibility is crucial. Traditional therapy for CAS involved drills with many repetitions of just a few words or phrases. Although this strategy resulted in improved accuracy on those specific utterances, the learning did not generalize to other words or phrases. SLPs now understand that, while intensive practice is vital for children with CAS, practice must include varied targets and contexts in order to train the speech motor planning system to develop motor programs for novel utterances as well as those that have been drilled.

When the speech sound disorder is cognitive-linguistic, the focus of therapy is on helping the child to understand the contrastive elements in their language(s). They need to learn, for example, that /b/ and /p/ are different phonemes (in English and many other languages) and that "stuck" and "tuck" and "tusk" are different words (in English) – the /s/ changes the meaning, not only due to its sheer presence but also based upon where in the word it occurs.

Fortunately, many intervention programs, strategies, and materials exist to assist speech-language pathologists in providing the appropriate types of therapy for children with different speech sound disorders. The challenge is that many of these are only available in a few languages.

Fluency Disorders

Distinguishing Typical and Atypical Disfluencies

As noted above, fluency refers to the smooth production of connected speech. All speakers, both children and adults, are disfluent sometimes. Furthermore, it is not unusual for children to go through a period of "normal disfluency" at about age 3 (Ambrose & Yairi, 1999), during which their speech temporarily becomes less smooth, more hesitant, and more repetitive. Disfluent behaviors that are considered to be normal (in children or adults) are typically brief (1/2 s or less) repetitions of sounds, syllables, or short words, such as "N-no, no; I don't think so" (Guitar & Conture, 2013). Occasional pauses, hesitations, or fillers (such as "um" in English, "euh" in French, "este" in Spanish) are also normal. These disfluencies usually occur when the child (or adult) is:

- Tired
- Excited about something
- Trying to express a complex idea
- Engaged in a question-answer interchange
- Getting little feedback or negative feedback from the listener

The factors that determine whether a child's disfluencies are typical or atypical include:

- Frequency (how often they happen)
- Duration (how long they last)
- Response/attitude (how the child appears to feel about the disfluencies; how she reacts when they occur)

(Guitar & Conture, 2013)

Stuttering

Stuttering (atypical disfluency) is diagnosed when some of the following are noted:

- Repetitions, tense pauses, or fillers occur on 3% (mild) to 10% or more (moderate to severe) of the words the child attempts.
- Sounds are occasionally (mild) or frequently (moderate to severe) prolonged.
- Complete blocks occur (moderate to severe) – little or no sound comes out despite effort.
- Repetitions, prolongations, blocks, or hesitations last ½–1 s (mild) or longer (moderate to severe).

- The child exhibits some concern (mild), frustration, embarrassment, and/or fear of speaking (moderate to severe) (Guitar & Conture, 2013).

Approximately 2% of children between the ages of 3 and 10 years stutter (prevalence; ASHA Practice Portal, 2016 - http://www.asha.org/Practice-Portal/Clinical-Topics/Childhood-Fluency-Disorders/ accessed 7/24/16). Stuttering often results in negative perceptions of the child, even by adults as well as by peers, who may belittle or tease the stutterer, further increasing the anxiety associated with oral communication.

Risk Factors The risk of a child becoming a chronic stutterer is increased when the following factors are present:

- There is a family history of chronic stuttering.
- The child is male.
- The stuttering begins after age 3.
- The child has a speech delay or disorder (see above).
- The child has a language delay or disorder (see Chapters 5–7).
- The stuttering has persisted for 6 months or more.
- The stuttering is not decreasing over time.

Course of Treatment It is very important to seek assistance as soon as possible for a child who is stuttering. In many cases, parent counseling is sufficient to ensure that newly emergent mild stuttering will decrease and eventually cease. Recommendations made to parents to alleviate their children's stuttering include the following:

- Modeling slower, more relaxed speech
- Decreasing the number of questions they ask the child and the amount of communication pressure that they put on her
- Communicating verbally and nonverbally that the child has the parents' and other family members' full attention when he is speaking:
  - Don't interrupt.
  - Take turns talking to be sure the child has opportunities to express himself.
  - Look at the child's face or at what he is looking at while he is talking.
  - Acknowledge what the child has said ("Oh, yes, that water is very cold.").
  - Set aside one-on-one times, ideally multiple times per week, when the child has the full attention of an important adult during a joint activity, during which he may or may not talk; no communication pressure. The adult should talk slowly and in a relaxed way, "like Mr. Rogers," during this activity (Guitar & Conture, 2013).

A speech-language pathologist with experience in working with children who stutter will be able to guide the parents in implementing these strategies, to assess the child to determine whether she also needs individual speech-language intervention, and to provide an appropriate course of treatment if so.

Cluttering

Cluttering is a different type of fluency disorder, which may or may not accompany stuttering or other childhood communication disorders, in which the child speaks too rapidly or with an uneven rate, sometimes resulting in leaving out syllables or even whole words. Typical disfluencies (see above) may also occur. Unlike children who stutter, children who clutter often appear to be unaware of their speech disorder. Therefore, they are less likely to notice listeners' difficulties and to try to clarify when they are not understood. The exact prevalence of cluttering – alone or in conjunction with other childhood communication disorders – is not established (ASHA Practice Portal Childhood Fluency Disorders http://www.asha.org/Practice-Portal/Clinical-Topics/Childhood-Fluency-Disorders/ accessed 7/24/16).

Voice Disorders

Not only is one's voice key to being able to express one's thoughts and needs, but the quality, tone, and intensity of the voice are also critical components of a person's identity. As with speech sound disorders and stuttering, children with voice disorders are often viewed more negatively both by their teachers and by their peers. The incidence of voice disorders in children has been estimated to range from 1 to 23%; best guesses at prevalence vary from 6% to 9%. The long-term vocal and social consequences of such conditions are largely unknown.

The sound of the voice depends on adequate respiration (i.e., properly functioning lungs), phonation (i.e., properly functioning larynx and vocal folds), and resonance (i.e., a properly functioning pharynx and vocal tract). If respiration is weak, the voice may be too quiet or the person may not be able to produce a whole phrase or sentence on one breath. If the vocal folds are physically different due to damage or a growth, or physiologically impaired due to weakness or incoordination, the voice will be breathy, quiet, strident, harsh, hoarse, or otherwise auditorily insufficient or displeasing to the ear (Hooper, 2004). If air leaks into the nasal cavity at inappropriate times due to cleft palate or another type of velopharyngeal insufficiency, the person's speech will be hypernasal, and it will be difficult for the listener to discern the intended consonant and vowel sounds (Hooper, 2004). In extreme cases, the person may not be able to speak audibly at all.

The primary cause of voice disorders in children is hyperfunction, i.e., overuse/abuse of the voice via yelling, loud and/or prolonged talking (especially in noisy situations), and/or excessive throat clearing or coughing. This typically results in hoarseness, with 45–80% of children also exhibiting vocal nodules (growths on the vocal folds) (Hooper, 2004). Hearing problems, allergies, asthma, upper respiratory tract infections, smoking, and gastroesophageal reflux may be contributory factors. Speech and language disorders also may coexist with voice disorders.

Course of Treatment Voice disorders in children are likely to become worse if left untreated. Treatment approaches for voice disorders, in descending order of invasiveness, include surgery, other medical intervention, direct voice therapy, and vocal hygiene programs. Often a combination of interventions is most appropriate.

Vocal hygiene programs may be effectively provided preventatively to groups of schoolchildren, or they may involve short periods of training for children who already have voice disorders and their parents, with carry-over then continuing in the home and at school. Such programs may involve child-level instruction about anatomy and physiology via pictures or videos, creative craft projects (e.g., a model larynx), peer critiquing, role playing/play acting, monitoring charts, and props such as water bottles to improve hydration (Von Berg & McFarlane, 2002). If need be, longer-term individual therapy can be provided. Components include general awareness, identification of overuse behaviors and how to change them, practice of healthy vocal production, and generalization activities. It is typically effective.

Medical interventions may include treatment for contributory factors (such as allergies, asthma, upper respiratory tract infections, and gastroesophageal reflux) or even surgery in more severe cases, to remove a growth (polyp, cyst, etc.) that is interfering with proper vocal function. However, surgery is usually not necessary/appropriate for vocal nodules; voice therapy is typically sufficient to reduce the size of the nodules (Hooper, 2004).

Cultural-Linguistic Considerations in the Development of Speech

The language(s) to which a child is exposed influences the development of speech and the identification, assessment, and treatment of speech disorders and should be considered in your screening of a child's speech. For example, the frequency of various types of speech sounds and their contrastive function in the native language(s) influences their order of acquisition among children. The formant frequencies (harmonics) of even the basic [a], [i] ("ee"), and [u] vowels differ from language to language, even when gender, age, weight, and height are controlled (Andrianopoulos, Darrow & Chen, 2001). Resonance (the "tone" of the voice) expectations also differ from one language group to another. For instance, some American dialects are significantly more nasal than others. Similarly, in some American age cohorts, vocal fry (the use of extremely low pitch) is expected in certain contexts for those who wish to be accepted as part of the "in group."

Cultural considerations must also be taken into account. Attitudes and expectations about speech clarity and fluency and about vocal quality vary widely from one cultural group to another. In addition, responses to disabilities – including communication disorders – differ significantly among different ethnic groups and may include shame or even rejection of the person with the impairment. In these cases, an additional responsibility is placed upon the primary healthcare provider, to increase understanding and acceptance of the communication condition before any formal assessment or intervention can be considered.

References

Ambrose, N. G., & Yairi, E. (1999). Normative disfluency data for early childhood stuttering. *Journal of Speech, Language and Hearing Research, 42*, 895–909.
American Speech-Language-Hearing Association (n.d.). Fluency Disorders in Childhood (Practice Portal). Retrieved from http://www.asha.org/Practice-Portal/Clinical-Topics/Childhood-Fluency-Disorders.
Andrianopoulos, M. V., Darrow, K., & Chen, J. (2001). Multimodal standardization of voice among four multicultural populations formant structures. *Journal of Voice, 15*(1), 61–77.
Black, L. I., Vahratian, A., & Hoffman, H. J. (2015). *Communication disorders and use of intervention services among children aged 3–17 years: United States, 2012 NCHS Data Brief.* Hyattsville, MD: National Center for Health Statistics.
Crelin, E. (1987). *The human vocal tract*. New York: Vantage.
Guitar, B., & Conture, E. (2013). *To the pediatrician*. Memphis, TN: Stuttering Foundation of America.
Hooper, C. R. (2004). Treatment of voice disorders in children. *Language Speech and Hearing Services in the Schools, 35*, 320–326.
Lewis, B. A., & Freebairn, L. A. (1992). Residual effects of preschool phonology disorders in grade school, adolescence, and adulthood. *Journal of Speech and Hearing Research, 35*, 819–831.
Messner, A. H., & Lalakea, M. L. (2002). The effect of ankyloglossia on speech in children. *Otolaryngology - Head and Neck Surgery, 127*(6), 539–545.
Miller, J. F., & Leddy, M. (1998). Down syndrome: The impact of speech production on language production. In R. Paul (Ed.), *Exploring the speech-language connection* (pp. 139–162). Baltimore, MD: Brookes.
Pennington, L., Parker, N. K., Kelly, H., & Miller, N. (2016). *Speech therapy for children with dysarthria acquired before three years of age* (Review). The Cochrane Library, 7. doi:10.1002/14651858.CD006937.pub3.
Rupela, V., & Manjula, R. (2007). Phonotactic patterns in the speech of children with Down syndrome. *Clinical Linguistics and Phonetics, 21*(8), 605–622.
Swift, E., & Rosin, P. (1990). A remediation sequence to improve speech intelligibility for students with Down syndrome. *Language, Speech and Hearing Services in Schools, 21*, 140–146.
Von Berg, S., & McFarlane, S. C. (2002). A collaborative approach to the diagnosis and treatment of child voice disorders. *ASHA Special Interest Division #3 Newsletter: Voice and Voice Disorders* (March), 19–21.

Other Resources

www.apraxia-kids.org
www.stutteringhelp.org

Chapter 9
Children with Hearing Loss

Introduction

Hearing loss is a complex condition that impacts all ages and has a variety of causes and conditions. It can be inherited or acquired, and understanding both the etiology and the impact has important implications for practitioners who are providing clinical management and support for children with hearing loss and their families. The American College of Medical Genetics and Genomics has guidelines for the clinical evaluation and etiologic diagnosis of hearing loss which is a helpful resource for providers (Alfred et al., 2014). The focus of this chapter is on hearing loss in children.

A recent report by the World Health Organization (WHO) on the status of childhood hearing loss, its causes and impact, indicates that 60% of childhood hearing loss could be prevented (ASHA, 2016). Nearly 10% of the 360 million people in the world's population who live with a hearing loss are children living in low- and middle-income countries. An estimated 40% of those with hearing loss are associated with genetic causes, while 60% are associated with infections (e.g., measles, mumps, rubella, and meningitis), birth complications, and ototoxic medication use in expecting mothers and newborns. The WHO believes that childhood hearing loss could be reduced with such preventive measures as immunizations, good hygiene, improved maternal and child health practices, and avoidance of ototoxic drugs. The WHO report highlights the importance of early identification and intervention and the impact of unaddressed hearing loss.

In an effort to address early identification of hearing loss, by 2011 almost 98% of infants born in the USA were screened shortly after birth (Centers for Disease Control and Prevention, 2013). Importantly, however, some mild, frequency-specific, late-onset, or progressive hearing losses may not be identified during this universal newborn hearing period. Notably, close to 15% of school-age children in the USA exhibit some level/type of hearing loss (Niskar et al., 1998). Further,

P. A. Prelock, T. L. Hutchins, *Clinical Guide to Assessment and Treatment of Communication Disorders*, Best Practices in Child and Adolescent Behavioral Health Care, https://doi.org/10.1007/978-3-319-93203-3_9

nearly 40% of children with hearing loss have secondary or concomitant conditions, so their function is impacted not only by hearing but other diagnoses (Gallaudet Research Institute, 2011). Hearing, therefore, is a critical function to screen, assess, and support on an ongoing basis with its crucial role in daily communication, function, and participation.

This chapter briefly describes the development of normal hearing, the anatomy of the auditory system, the hearing impairments primary healthcare providers are likely to see and the impact on communication, and the common approaches to assessing hearing in children. The chapter ends with an explanation of some preventive steps to hearing loss as well as intervention strategies that can be used to enhance auditory function, communication, and learning success.

Development of Normal Hearing

Understanding the auditory development of children is important as it has an impact on learning and long-term function. Auditory development begins in the fetal period with a 20-week-old fetus responding with an increased heart rate when sound is presented (Hedge, 2010). As newborns, infants open or blink their eyes in response to sound. A startle response to sound is often seen with sudden arm and leg movements as well as a cease of such movement or crying when sound is introduced. At 3 months, infants respond to their mother's voice and turn their head toward sound by 3–4 months with greater precision reflecting improved sound localization as they approach their sixth and seventh months.

In normal hearing sound is conducted in two ways, through air conduction and bone conduction. In air conduction sound is transmitted through air, and sound waves strike the ear drum which are transmitted to the three bones of the middle ear (called the ossicular chain). This moves the fluids of the inner ear causing vibrations on the basilar membrane of the cochlea. The hair cells of the cochlea are connected to the acoustic nerve, and, when stimulated by these vibrations, sound is carried to the brain. In contrast, sound carried through bone conduction is transmitted through the vibrations of the skull and the three bones of the middle ear, which causes movement of the inner ear fluids and subsequent stimulation of the acoustic nerve (Hedge, 2010).

Typically, we hear our own voice through both air and bone conduction. A young and healthy individual can hear sounds in the frequency (i.e., the number of times a cycle of vibration repeats itself within a second) of 20 Hz to 20,000Hz. Adults, however, don't hear as well as children and youth because of changes in the hearing mechanism with exposure to noise, the general aging process, and an individual's auditory health. Importantly, speech is produced in the frequency range of 100 HZ to 5000Hz – the important range for communication.

Anatomy of the Auditory System

Hearing is made possible by the important structures for hearing: the ear, acoustic nerve, and auditory areas of the brain. The outer ear (auricle or pinna) helps localize sounds, and the external auditory canal secretes wax (cerumen) to trap small insects or other debris that might enter the middle ear. The middle ear is filled with air and includes the tympanic membrane (eardrum), the ossicular chain (three small bones), and the eustachian tube. The tympanic membrane separates the middle and outer ears and can be easily damaged by sudden pressure changes that could rupture the membrane. Although it often heals spontaneously, damage can leave tissue that is scarred, reducing mobility of the membrane.

The ossicular chain includes the malleus, incus, and stapes (stirrup). The malleus is the first and largest of the three bones and looks like a hammer. One end is attached to the tympanic membrane so vibrations of the membrane are transmitted to the malleus. The malleus is also attached to the second bone, the incus which is attached to the third bone or stapes which is inserted into a small opening (oval window) leading to the inner ear (Hedge, 2010). The three bones are efficient sound transmitters. The eustachian tube (or auditory tube) connects the middle ear with the nasopharynx or opening to the nasal passage. The eustachian tube helps maintain equal air pressure within and outside the middle ear and provides a way of clearing the middle ear space of any debris or fluid.

The inner ear is more complex and begins with the oval window and interconnecting tunnels or labyrinths filled with fluid that are housed in the temporal bone. Two structures within the inner ear that have unrelated functions are the vestibular system and the cochlea. The vestibular system contains three semicircular canals that have a role in balance, body position, and movement. The cochlea is the more important structure for hearing. It is a snail-shaped coiled tunnel filled with fluid. It has a basilar membrane and contains the organs of Corti which bathes in the fluid and has thousands of hair cells that respond to sound.

The acoustic nerve (cranial nerve VIII) is a bundle of neurons with a vestibular branch and an auditory or acoustic branch which connects to the hair cells of the cochlea and is concerned with sound transmission. It carries electrical sound impulses from the cochlea to the brain (Hedge, 2010).

Hearing Impairment in Children and the Impact on Communication

Impairments in hearing have major influences on a child's health and education. Although hearing loss is often associated with aging, all ages are impacted as it has a notable social impact. Hearing loss can be mild with little to no impact on

Table 9.1 Categories and range of hearing loss for children and likely impact on oral communication

Categories of hearing loss	Decibel (dB) level and range	Likely impact
Normal	Up to 15 dB	It is important to assess the hearing of all children with a communication disorder to ensure hearing is not part of the challenge they are experiencing
Mild	16–40 dB	Children may have difficulty hearing faint speech or speech at a distance, which could cause a delay in their language
Moderate	41–55 dB	Children with a loss in this range will experience difficulty acquiring speech and language delay, have speech sound production problems, and have problems following conversation
Moderately Severe	56–70 dB	Children will be unable to hear without amplification of some kind
Severe	71–90 dB	Children will have difficulty hearing amplified speech, impacting their learning and ability to produce intelligible oral communication
Profound	91+ dB	Children with hearing in this range are considered deaf; thus, hearing will not have a significant role in their learning or understanding and producing oral communication

Adapted from Hedge (2010, p. 502)

communication or profound with significant problems in receptive and expressive language and speech sound production. Table 9.1 summarizes the categories of hearing loss a provider will see in children, the decibel (a basic unit of measurement for intensity or what we experience as loudness) level and range for children with normal hearing and hearing loss, and the likely impact of the hearing loss on the understanding and use of speech and language or oral communication.

Hearing disorders are also classified into those which lead to conductive hearing loss, sensorineural hearing loss, both conductive and sensorineural loss, and two other special types of impairment known as auditory processing disorder and auditory neuropathy. Table 9.2 defines these hearing impairment types and briefly highlights the likely causes. The two most common causes of conductive loss, however, which practitioners are most likely to see in children are otitis media and cholesteatoma. The problems of otitis media are particularly relevant for providers as it is a common occurrence with nearly 95% of children affected at least once in childhood and many children having recurrent episodes. It is important to understand that this frequent occurrence will likely have an impact on a child's speech and language development as the peak time for ear infections is the first 2 years or life. Otitis media seems to be more common in boys than girls, but the seasons when both sexes are most affected is winter and spring. Children with Down syndrome or cleft palate as well as Native American children are particularly at risk for ear infections (Hedge, 2010). The significant increase in reported infections has been attributed to an increased percentage of children attending day care where such infections are commonly transmitted (Bess & Humes, 2008).

Table 9.2 Types and causes of hearing impairment

Type of hearing impairment	Definition	Causes
Conductive hearing loss	Diminished conduction of sound to the middle or inner ear	Abnormalities in the external auditory canal, eardrum, or ossicular chain caused by birth defects, diseases, and foreign bodies that block the external canal Aural atresia=>external ear canal (EEC) completely closed Stenosis=>EEC is very narrow External otitis=>infection often seen in swimmers causing a swelling of the canal tissue Bony growths or tumors=>block the EEC Otitis media=>middle ear (ME) effusion or an infection frequently associated with upper respiratory infections Serous ME inflamed and filled with fluid as eustachian tube is blocked Acute sudden onset of fluid and pus due to infection Chronic tympanic membrane is ruptured with or without ME disease Cholesteatoma=>skin growth occurring in the ME behind the eardrum; often as a result of poor eustachian tube function and ME infection
Sensorineural hearing loss	Hair cells in the cochlea or acoustic nerve are damaged, keeping the brain from receiving sound impulses	Ototoxic drugs (e.g., antibiotics of the "mycin" family) taken prenatally, esp. during gestation week 6 or 7 damage the cochlea of the fetus Sustained exposure to noise (e.g., loud music, firecrackers, explosives, noisy toys) damage the cochlear hair cells Infections, such as meningitis and maternal rubella, attack the inner ear Birth defects, such as those associated with the development of the cochlea or the acoustic nerve, syphilis contracted from the mother, or anoxia during delivery impact hearing A tumor (acoustic neuroma) occurs on rare occasions and interferes with nerve conduction of sound
Mixed hearing loss	Both the middle and inner ear are functioning poorly	Any of the conditions or combination of conditions noted for conductive and sensorineural hearing loss
Auditory processing disorders (formerly called central auditory processing disorders, CAPD)	Affect the central auditory system of 2–3% of children so that they have difficulty segmenting and sequencing sounds, particularly in noise or when input is distorted	Lesions in the central auditory systems, although not always evident in children
Auditory neuropathy spectrum disorder	Normal or near normal cochlear hair cell function but abnormal or absent acoustic nerve response	Syndromic, non-syndromic, or mitochondrial genetic factors

It should be noted that auditory processing disorder (APD) is a controversial topic in the discipline but has been reported as impacting a child's academic performance. Children with APD may have symptoms that overlap with children with autism spectrum disorder (ASD) or learning disorders (LD) as they will struggle with sound localization and direction following. Auditory neuropathy spectrum disorder (ANSD) is a relatively new term with its associated controversy as some suggest it should be differentiated from sensorineural hearing loss by the location of the pathology (spiral ganglion cells vs. hair cells) and more aptly called a neural hearing loss. Usually a child with ANSD will have adequate hair cell function in the cochlea and poor acoustic nerve function resulting in difficulties hearing in noise and inconsistent speech perception performance (Rance, Beer, Cone-Wesson, & Shepherd, 1999; Starr, Picton, Hood, & Berlin, 1996). The reported incidence of ANSD is more than 13% in children with severe-profound hearing loss (Sanyebhaa, Kabel, Sammy, & Elbadry, 2009). Of the children impacted by ANSD, 40% have a genetic basis (Clarin, 2015) with the greatest incidence occurring as the result of specific syndromes or mitochondrial genetic causes (Manchaiah, Zhao, Danesh, & Duprey, 2011).

The overall impact of hearing loss on a child's speech production, language development, vocal tone, and resonance quality is significant. It is important to understand this impact when supporting a child and family so that the child has full access to social and academic opportunities. Table 9.3 outlines the types of communication disorders children with a hearing loss are likely to experience.

Table 9.3 Types of speech, voice, resonance, language, and social cognition disorders common in children with hearing loss

Type of disorder	Characteristics	Examples
Speech	Sounds produced in the back of the mouth often omitted as they are more difficult to see	"du" for "duck"
	Omission of sounds in blends	"sar" for "star"
	Distort most consonants	[f, sh, th, ch]
	Substitute one sound for another	[b] for [p]
Voice	Breathy and harsh High pitch and unpredictable loudness	Voices sounds "throaty" Often because of the tension in the vocal folds
Resonance	Flat and monotonous	Lacks normal rhythm or speech; sounds disconnected
Language	Difficulty with grammar and sentence structure Omit grammatical morphemes Written language often shows similar problems as seen in oral language	Passive, compound, and embedded sentences are challenging Plural and possessive "s" Progressive "ing" Past tense "ed"
Social cognition	Difficulty understanding nonliteral language, humor, and the mental states of self vs. others	Jokes, sarcastic remarks, false beliefs

Hearing Assessment in Children

When there is concern about a hearing loss, a referral to an audiologist should occur as soon as possible. Being the expert in hearing and its disorders, an audiologist will work with a child and family to complete a comprehensive assessment, share results, and answer questions. There are several components to the testing the audiologist conducts, the most common being *pure tone audiometry*. Using an electronic instrument (audiometer) that presents sounds of varying intensity and pitches, the audiologist will test a child's sensitivity to "pure tones" or the sounds of specific frequencies. *Speech audiometry* might also be done as the pure tone testing doesn't tell the audiologist how well a child interprets speech sounds or discriminates between them. Another measurement is *acoustic immittance* which does not require the child to actively respond to any signals or speech. Instead a sound stimulus goes directly to the peripheral or central hearing mechanism through a transfer of acoustic energy (Bess & Humes, 2008; Martin & Clark, 2008). It is effective in identifying middle ear problems.

To address more inner ear problems without requiring a child to actively participate, *evoked otoacoustic emissions* can be obtained to determine how effectively the outer hair cells of the cochlea are functioning. *Electrophysiological audiometry* is also used to measure the brain's response to sound, including signals from the cochlea, acoustic nerve, and auditory centers of the brain. Abnormal patterns of electrical impulses can indicate hearing loss. *Auditory brainstem response* (ABR) identifies electrical activity in the acoustic nerve, while *electrocochleography* identifies electrical activity in the cochlea (Hedge, 2010). More advanced audiological tests are used to assess auditory processing disorders such as *dichotic listening tests* (stimuli presented to competing ears) or *binaural integration* (splitting the presentation of syllables from multisyllabic words to one ear and then the other).

Assessing the hearing of infants and young children is crucial because of the impact of hearing and hearing loss on language acquisition and the importance of early intervention. Although traditional audiometry will not typically work for young children, *behavioral observation audiometry* can be used. This approach tests the reflexive response of young children to sound (noise makers, calling the infant's name) and can be used for infants, birth to 6 months. For older infants, sound localization can be used where the audiologist looks for the child to turn their head in the direction of the sound heard. Some children between 6 and 30 months are able to be conditioned to wear headphones and respond to the pure tones presented through the headphones but require *conditioned play audiometry* where they learn to put a block in a container every time they hear a sound.

Supporting Hearing and Communication in Children

Hearing screening is a critical part of the care that should be provided to all children as part of their regular care, and it is particularly important for children with disabilities. Universal newborn hearing screening is recommended by the Joint

Committee on Infant Hearing (JCIH, 2007) and the NIDCD (1993), and guidelines are provided by the American Speech-Language-Hearing Association (1997). Although all states and public schools have their own policies on hearing screening and many participate in the Universal Newborn Hearing Screening Program, it is critical to screen hearing as early as possible to begin early intervention for children with hearing loss. Often, hearing screenings for children take place in early childhood, school, community or medical settings, or audiology clinics.

Since hearing is so crucial to language acquisition, sound production, and comprehension, as well as monitoring our speech production, hearing assessment, follow-up, and intervention are key to a child's success in school and in their community. The age of hearing loss is important as a congenital loss appears to have a greater impact than one sustained as an adult. Also, children who acquire language before their hearing loss do better than those who acquire a hearing loss before speech develops. Degree of hearing loss is also an important consideration as a more severe or profound loss will have a greater impact on language acquisition. Importantly, though, children who are deaf may not be considered to have a communication disorder because many acquire American Sign Language (ASL) with the help of parents and educators of the deaf which allows them to be efficient communicators. That said, it has been estimated that 95% of children with hearing loss are born to hearing parents who, even when trained early in the use of sign to augment communication, lack fluency in sign. This places children at risk for restricted access to language and language socialization.

For those children born with a bilateral, severe to profound hearing loss and who are unlikely to receive notable benefit from hearing aids, the standard of care has become cochlear implantation (Beer et al., 2014; Sarant & Garrard, 2014). A cochlear implant bypasses the damaged inner ear and uses an electrode array to stimulate the acoustic nerve, facilitating the brain's capacity to process sound (O'Donoghue, Nikolopoulos & Archbold, 2000). Although a cochlear implant does not restore hearing, if a child receives an implant by age 2, they are usually able to understand and produce spoken language with intense speech and language intervention. They are also able to enter a typical educational setting by first grade. Children with cochlear implants will show better oral language acquisition than those who don't have an implant. Their speech and language skills as well as their literacy skills, however, are usually behind those of their peers (Montgomery, Magimairaj, & Finney, 2010; Nittrouer, Caldwell, & Holloman, 2012). Theory of mind and more broadly social cognition skills are also delayed in children who are deaf or hard of hearing and have hearing parents (Peterson & Wellman, 2009; Peterson, Wellman, & Liu, 2005).

Habilitation is the step taken by audiologists, speech-language pathologists, and educators or the deaf and hard of hearing to lessen the impact of a child's hearing impairment. The goal of habilitation is to emphasize function and full participation of the child. The audiologist is responsible for aural rehabilitation which includes an evaluation of hearing loss, assessment of communication needs and hearing aid fittings, training in hearing aid use, and counseling the child and family. For children with hearing impairment, the speech-language pathologist works on the child's speech and language skills and helps to address their problems with voice, speech, rhythm, language, and socialization. The educator of the deaf helps to teach the child in the academic arena and incorporates other methods of communication like ASL. Children with hearing loss often learn to speech read by watching the movement of a speaker's articulators to help them understand oral language. Assistive listening devices are also used for watching television, talking on the phone, etc. Further, FM (frequency modulation) systems are used in the educational environment to provide optimal access to instruction and learning. FM systems also allow teachers to talk into a microphone which transmits the teacher's voice directly to the hearing aid of a child with a hearing loss. Importantly, though, parent training will be crucial to the communication and social and learning success of children with hearing loss.

Summary

It is important that providers understand the importance of hearing, its development, and the impact of its loss on the speech, language, and learning of children. "Failure to detect congenital or acquired hearing loss in children may result in lifelong deficits in speech and language acquisition, poor academic performance, personal-social maladjustments, and emotional difficulties" (Harlor & Bower, 2009, p. 1253). The impact of hearing loss is far reaching and does not have to be severe to impact a child's ability to access auditory-based classroom instruction. Newborn hearing screening is certainly an excellent first step in identifying hearing loss early on, but a plan must be in place for regular hearing screenings and follow-up. Primary healthcare providers should have an ongoing connection with an audiologist for assessment and consultation and should ensure that families have access to a speech-language pathologist to support appropriate interventions that are responsive to the varying cultural contexts for deafness and hearing.

Some resources providers might find useful can be found at the following links:

- http://www.asha.org/Practice-Portal/Professional-Issues/Childhood-Hearing-Screening/
- http://www.asha.org/buds/
- http://podcast.asha.org/episode-14-protecting-the-hearing-of-the-young-transcript/
- http://www.nidcd.nih.gov/health/hearing/pages/commopt.aspx
- http://research.gallaudet.edu/Demographics/deaf-US.php
- American Academy of Audiology Task Force. (2011). *Childhood hearing screening guidelines*. Retrieved from www.audiology.org/publications-resources/document-library/pediatric-diagnostics
- American Speech-Language-Hearing Association. (2004). *Scope of practice in audiology*[Scope of practice]. Available from www.asha.org/policy

- American Speech-Language-Hearing Association. (2006). *Preferred Practice Patterns for the Profession of Audiology*[Preferred practice patterns]. Available from www.asha.org/policy
- http://pediatrics.aappublications.org/content/early/2013/03/18/peds.2013-0008.citation (2013 EI supplement to JCIH 2007)

References

Alfred, R. L., Arnos, K. S., Fox, M., Lin, J. W., Palmer, C. G., Pandja, A., et al. (2014). ACMG Guideline for the clinical evaluation and etiologic diagnosis of hearing loss. *Genetics in Medicine, 16*(4), 347–355.

American Speech Language Hearing Association. (June, 2016). 60 percent of childhood hearing loss is preventable. *The Asha Leader, 21*, 12. https://doi.org/10.1044/leader.NIB6.21062016.12

American Speech Language Hearing Association Audiological Assessment Panel. (1997). *Guidelines for audiologic screening*. Rockville, MD: Author.

Beer, J., Kronenberger, W. G., Castellanos, I., Colson, B. G., Henning, S. C., & Pisoni, D. B. (2014). Executive functioning skills in preschool children with cochlear implants. *Journal of Speech, Language and Hearing Research, 57*, 1521–1534.

Bess, F. H., & Humes, L. E. (2008). *Audiology: The fundamentals-4th edition*. Philadelphia, PA: Lippincott Williams & Wilkins.

Centers for Disease Control and Prevention. (2013). *Summary of 2011 national EHDI data*. Retrieved from www.cdc.gov/ncbddd/hearingloss/2011-data/2011_ehdi_hsfs_summary_a.pdf.

Clarin, G. (2015). Auditory nerve pathway (Chapter 8). In *A resource guide early hearing screening and intervention*. MCHAM e-book.

Gallaudet Research Institute. (April, 2011). *Regional and National Summary Report of Data from the 2009-10 Annual Survey of Deaf and Hard of Hearing Children and Youth*. Washington, DC: GRI, Gallaudet University.

Harlor Jr., A. D., & Bower, C. (2009). Hearing assessment in infants and children: Recommendations beyond neonatal screening. *Pediatrics, 124*(4), 1252–1263.

Hedge, M. N. (2010). Audiology: Hearing and its disorders. In *Introduction to communicative disorders-4th edition* (pp. 487–529). Austin, TX: Pro-ed.

Joint Committee on Infant Hearing. (2007). Year 2007 position statement: Principles and guidelines for early hearing detection and intervention programs. *Pediatrics, 120*(4), 898–921.

Manchaiah, V. K. C., Zhao, F., Danesh, A. A., & Duprey, R. (2011). The genetic basis of auditory neuropathy spectrum disorder (ANSD). *International Journal of Pediatric Otorhinolaryngology, 75*, 151–158.

Martin, F. N., & Clark, J. G. (2008). *Introduction to audiology-10th edition*. Boston: Allyn & Bacon.

Montgomery, J. W., Magimairaj, B. M., & Finney, M. C. (2010). Working memory and specific language impairment: An update on the relation and perspectives on assessment and treatment. *American Journal of Speech-Language Pathology, 19*, 78–94.

National Institute on Deafness and Other Communication Disorders (NIDCD). (1993). *National Institutes of Health Consensus Statement: Early identification of hearing impairment in infants and young children*. Bethesda, MD: Author.

Niskar, A. S., Kieszak, S. M., Holmes, A., Esteban, E., Rubin, C., & Brody, D. J. (1998). Prevalence of hearing loss among children 6 to 19 years of age. *Journal of the American Medical Association, 279*(14), 1071–1075.

Nittrouer, S., Caldwell, A., & Holloman, C. (2012). Measuring what matters: Effectively predicting language and literacy in children with cochlear implants. *International Journal of Pediatric Otorhinolaryngology, 76*, 1148–1158.

O'Donoghue, G. M., Nikolopoulos, T. P., & Archbold, S. M. (2000). Determinants of speech perception in children after cochlear implantation. *The Lancet, 356*, 466–468.

Peterson, C. C., & Wellman, H. M. (2009). From fancy to reason: Scaling deaf children's theory of mind and pretence. *British Journal of Developmental Psychology, 27*, 297–310.

Peterson, C. C., Wellman, H. M., & Liu, D. (2005). Steps in theory of mind development for children with autism, deafness or typical development. *Child Development, 76*, 502–517.

Rance, G., Beer, D., Cone-Wesson, B., & Shepherd, R. (1999). Clinical findings for a group of infants and young children with auditory neuropathy. *Ear and Hearing, 20*, 238–252.

Sanyelbhaa, T. H., Kabel, A. H., Sammy, H., & Elbadry, M. (2009). Prevalence of auditory neuropathy (AN) among infants and young children with severe to profound hearing loss. *International Journal of Pediatric Otorhinolaryngology, 73*(7), 937–939.

Sarant, J., & Garrard, P. (2014). Parenting stress in parents of children with cochlear implants: Relationships among parent stress, child language, and unilateral versus bilateral implants. *Journal of Deaf Studies and Deaf Education, 19*, 85–106.

Starr, A., Picton, T., Hood, L. J., & Berlin, C. (1996). Auditory neuropathy. *Brain, 119*, 741–753.

Chapter 10
Children with Intellectual Disability

Introduction

More than one in seven US children have a behavioral, developmental, or mental disability (American Speech, Language, and Hearing Association, 2016). Developmental disabilities, a common occurrence, are usually severe, chronic, and identified in children 5 years and older and typically before 22 years of age. They are characterized by functional limitations in three or more areas of daily life activities such as receptive and expressive language, learning, mobility, self-care, and capacity for independent learning (Developmental Disabilities Assistance and Bill of Rights Act, 2000). The focus of this chapter is intellectual disabilities, one of several developmental disabilities children experience that impact their ability to communicate. With an onset prior to 18 years, children with intellectual disabilities have challenges in a variety of areas of cognitive function including learning, reasoning, and problem-solving (American Association on Intellectual and Developmental Disabilities; AAIDD, 2013a, b). Often, these challenges are accompanied by difficulties in understanding and producing verbal or even gestural messages, depending on the significance of their cognitive limitations. They also experience challenges in their adaptive functioning, which relates to their conceptual understanding of daily events and the personal and social skills needed to adapt to those events. Again, difficulty communicating will compromise a child's ability to understand what might be expected in a typical routine or how to initiate interactions and engage socially in an age appropriate manner.

Our understanding of intellectual disability (ID) has evolved over the years as a reflection of a number of changes made to both the social and legal advancements observed for those affected and their families. In the USA, intervention and support have moved from an institutional approach to a more inclusive, community-based approach with an emphasis on self-advocacy and self-determination and an increased focus on the communication rights of persons with ID (NJC,

P. A. Prelock, T. L. Hutchins, *Clinical Guide to Assessment and Treatment of Communication Disorders*, Best Practices in Child and Adolescent Behavioral Health Care, https://doi.org/10.1007/978-3-319-93203-3_10

1992; Brady et al., 2016). Previously, children with ID were called mentally retarded with intellectual capacity as the defining feature. More recently, a recognition of the relative strengths of the individual with intellectual challenges is important to consider as well as their adaptive functioning (Schalock, Luckasson, & Shorgren, 2007). Fortunately, this more inclusive definition recognizes the importance of balancing a child's limitations with their relative skills so that the supports provided maximize a child's individual abilities without focusing solely on what they can't do.

In the *Diagnostic and Statistical Manual of Mental Disorders* (*DSM-5*; American Psychiatric Association [APA], 2013), ID is defined in a manner similar to the AAIDD definition while expanding the definition to include severity levels (i.e., mild, moderate, severe, and profound). It also considers a child's adaptive functioning in three domains: conceptual, social, and practical. Under the new AAIDD and DSM-5 definitions of ID, limitations in adaptive functions are a requirement for diagnosis. The expanded definitions fit well with the World Health Organization's (WHO, 2001) *International Classification of Functioning, Disability and Health* (ICF) and the *ICF Children and Youth Version* (WHO, 2007) explanation for ID that recognizes not only impairments in body functions and structures but activity and participation limitations. Levels of support are also defined, including (1) *intermittent*, supports are used as needed, so they may be episodic or short term or occur during transitions such as school to work or a job loss; (2) *limited*, supports are more consistently needed over time and require fewer staff and less cost than higher levels of support; (3) *extensive*, supports are provided on a regular or daily basis and are long term and not time limited with some involvement in the child's living environments (e.g., employment, residential); and (4) *pervasive*, supports are constant, high-intensity, and provided in all environments.

Prevalence

Unfortunately, because researchers do not operationalize ID in the same manner, prevalence numbers (those living with ID in a given period) are complicated and should be interpreted with caution. In some cases, an intelligence quotient (IQ) cutoff score is used to make a diagnosis, while in other cases there is a more qualitative assessment of function such as identified limitations in adaptive and intellectual function. With these differences in mind, there are several reports of varying prevalence rates for both international and US samples. In a meta-analysis of international studies, the prevalence of ID in children and adolescents was 1.83% (Maulik, Mascarenhas, Mathers, Dua, & Saxena, 2011) with a range from 0.22% to 1.55% in a follow-up study (McKenzie, Milton, Smith & Ouellette-Kuntz, 2016). Notably, the ratio of females to males revealed 4–10 females for every 10 males with an ID (Maulik et al., 2011; Maulik, Mascarenhas, Mathers, Dua, & Saxena, 2013).

For US children under 18 years of age, ID prevalence was identified as 0.5% in the 2006–2010 National Health Interview Survey (Schieve et al., 2012) although the percent was much higher (5.8%) for children 2–17 years of age in the 2009–2010 National Survey of Children with Special Healthcare Needs. For US children under 15 years of age, the 2010 Census Bureau revealed 0.4% had an ID (Brault, 2012). When examining 2014–2015 school year data and those served under the Individuals with Disabilities Education Act (Part B), the prevalence of ID for 3- to 5-year-olds was 0.12% and 0.62% for 6- to 21 years old (US Department of Education, 2015).

Causes

Intellectual disabilities are seen as a result of three primary causes: prenatal, perinatal, and postnatal. Prenatal causes are most often the result of genetic syndromes which account for about 45% of the intellectual disabilities healthcare providers are likely to see (Bashaw, Roizen & Lotrecchiano, 2013) with Down syndrome being the largest genetic cause, Fragile X being the largest inherited cause, and fetal alcohol being the largest environmental cause (www.asha.org/practice-portal). Perinatal causes are related to difficulties at birth such as anoxia. There are a number of postnatal causes, but most occur because of a traumatic brain injury, infections, seizure disorders, chronic social deprivations, or toxic metabolic conditions such as lead and mercury poisoning.

General Communication Difficulties in Children with ID

Children with ID who also experience speech and language disorders will likely have poorly developed phonology (speech sound production), syntax (grammar), morphology (aspects of language that provide additional meaning like pluralization and past tense), semantics (word meaning), and pragmatics (social use of language). See Chapter 2 in this book for additional information regarding these language concepts. Children with ID are likely to have varying levels of compromised receptive language function (comprehension of words spoken or read) and expressive language function (oral or written forms), and many will use multiple means to communicate including sign language, pictures, computer systems, and voice output devices. Because of their communication challenges, many will also experience behavioral and social problems.

Generally, language will be less complex and more concrete when compared to children without ID. Vocabulary will likely be limited, and only simple instructions and gestures may be understood. Expressive language may be characterized more by gestures, facial expressions, signs, and other means of augmentative and alternative communication than by intelligible, complex sentences and narrative discourse. With limited language comprehension and production, social skills are often immature, with poorly developed social judgment and decision-making and less attention to social cues and rules.

Co-occurring Conditions and Disorders with ID and Communication Impairments

There are a variety of conditions that can co-occur with children who have intellectual disabilities. Communication skills vary depending not only on severity of the disability but also the other co-occurring conditions or behavioral, social, and emotional factors that characterize the individual. The most common co-occurring conditions seen in childhood include but are not limited to autism spectrum disorders, cerebral palsy, Down syndrome, fetal alcohol syndrome, and Fragile X. Additionally, children with intellectual disability might also experience an anxiety disorder, attention deficit hyperactivity disorder, and depressive and bipolar disorder to name a few (APA, 2013). Table 10.1 presents a brief description of the likely communication difficulties for the most commonly occurring intellectual disabilities.

Table 10.1 Communication difficulties for commonly occurring ID[a]

Commonly occurring conditions with ID	Speech-language challenges	Other related communication challenges
Autism spectrum disorders	Echolalia; perseverative language use; delay or lack of spoken language; poor receptive language; difficulty with narrative discourse	Deficits in initiation of and response to joint attention; difficulties in social initiation and social referencing; some feeding problems
Cerebral palsy	Language disorders; childhood apraxia of speech; dysarthria	May have hearing loss; feeding and swallowing difficulties
Down syndrome	Speech and language production problems, with better receptive than expressive language; poor intelligibility of speech; syntax or grammar compromised more than semantics or word meaning; stuttering is common	Chronic otitis media, persistent conductive or sensorineural hearing loss; stronger social skills although difficulty with higher level skills like idioms and figurative language
Fetal alcohol syndrome	Speech and language delayed; receptive and expressive language challenges; problems with narrative discourse	Hearing loss; social communication difficulties
Fragile X	Speech and language delays, with grammar compromised more than vocabulary or receptive language; problems in fluency, articulation and oral motor skills; unintelligible connected speech	Social communication difficulties similar to those of children with autism

[a]See www.asha.org/practice-Portal/Clinical-Topics/Intellectual-Disability for additional information

Other Health Conditions

Notably, children with ID may have a greater incidence of health problems than those children without disabilities. Unfortunately, this is often due to poorer healthcare and a lack of understanding of the unique special healthcare needs for these special populations (Krahn, Hammond, & Turner, 2006; van Schrojenstein Lantman-de Valk & Noonan Walsh, 2008). Further, limitations in communication (Gentile, Cowan, & Smith, 2015) compromise the child's ability to talk about their health needs including describing pain, identifying the location of discomfort, and explaining the symptoms and the timeline of onset sensory issues such as hearing loss (Herer, 2012) and visual impairment (Warburg, 2001) which are particular areas of compromise for children with ID and require ongoing follow-up. Heart conditions (Patja, Molska, & Iivanainen, 2001), seizure activity (Oeseburg, Dijkstra, Groothoff, Reijneveld, & Jansen, 2011), and obesity (Rimmer, Yamaki, Lowry, Wang, & Vogel, 2010) are also common and require ongoing care. Unfortunately, the focus on ID in medical school is limited (Sullivan et al., 2011) but necessary if we wish to address health disparities and improve the quality of life for children with intellectual disabilities.

Assessment

The screening and assessment of children with or at risk for ID requires a team of professionals because of the likely challenges across developmental domains. The specific team members will depend on the individual needs of the child, but overall the team identifies both strengths and challenges in adaptive function and determines needed supports across the conceptual, practical, and social domains for learning. Families are important members of the assessment team as they provide critical and unique information about their children's strengths, challenges, and needs. They understand their children's communication needs, know the expected routines throughout the day, and value outcomes that ensure health, safety, independence, and the development of meaningful relationships for their children (Giangreco, 1990).

Most often, a child's intellectual capacity is assessed using a measure of intelligence, while an assessment of adaptive behavior provides a more comprehensive view of a child's capacity or potential to function in everyday life. There are skills children need to function in everyday life including the ability to use language to communicate, read, and learn information; tell time and understand money concepts; problem-solve in social situations; follow rules; connect with others; recognize and avoid dangerous situations; bathe, groom, and toilet independently; use transportation; follow schedules; use the telephone; and work. These skills require a basic understanding of concepts, social awareness, and practical skills to increase independence. There are several measures that are used to assess adaptive behavior including the *Vineland Adaptive Behavior Scale, Second Edition* (Sparrow, Cicchetti, & Balla, 2005) and the *Supports Intensity Scale* (AAIDD, 2013a, b).

The role of speech-language pathologists (SLPs) and audiologists is to screen the speech, language, and hearing skills of children with or at risk for ID. Following screening, a decision is made regarding the need for a more comprehensive assessment. Since communication impairments often co-occur for children with ID, it is important that they have a comprehensive assessment of their receptive and expressive language including an assessment of their hearing. Approaches to communication assessment must be culturally and linguistically sensitive and carefully selected depending on the severity of the disability. Accommodations would need to be made for any children with sensory or mobility challenges. Testing approaches would be modified to ensure a child's full potential was assessed.

Assessment will likely include both formal and informal measures. More formal testing is required to make a diagnosis of an ID and to determine whether a child is eligible for services. More informal testing is used to identify a child's relative strengths, developmental milestone achievements, and limitations across various developmental domains. Often, this includes parent informant measures, parent interviews, observations of the child in a variety of contexts, and elicited play tasks. Regardless of a child's age and ability level, a comprehensive assessment should be completed and include the following elements:

- Case history review of the child's educational, medical, and home status
- Interviews with caregivers, teachers, and others who spend time with the child on a regular basis
- Hearing, vision, motor, and cognitive examinations
- Assessment of the child's vocalizations, gesture use, speech sound and word production, fluency, and use of signs and pictures to communicate
- Assessment of independent play and play with peers
- Observation of social interactions and social communication with peers and adults
- Assessment of receptive and expressive language including listening, speaking, reading, and writing
- Examination of the child's oral motor and swallowing skills

This multifaceted approach to assessment is important to ensure the clinician has a comprehensive profile of the child's strengths and challenges. Additionally, the clinician would need to have an understanding of the child's community environment so that whatever supports are provided, they are aligned with the child's current cultural context. Ultimately, a comprehensive profile of a child's intellectual, adaptive, and communication strengths, challenges, and needs will lead to individualized supports designed to improve the child's quality of life. Findings from these assessments, however, should be considered in the context of findings from other professionals (e.g., developmental pediatrician, psychologist, special educator). Moreover, families should be the decision-makers about next steps and the priorities they have for their children's goals and objectives.

At times, it may be difficult to differentiate between ID and other developmental disorders (e.g., language disorders, hearing loss, autism) where communication problems can be mistakenly attributed to ID. It is important that clinicians are aware of the differentiating characteristics of a variety of developmental disabilities. If a physician is unclear about the specific diagnosis, a referral should be made to a team that specializes in the assessment of children with neurodevelopmental disabilities.

Service Eligibility

In the USA, children and adolescents with ID are eligible for SLP services because communication skills are necessary for effective functioning, regardless of age or cognitive ability. Fortunately, the eligibility rules for services have changed and now recognize that it is inappropriate to have a priori criteria (e.g., cognitive referencing) to determine who may or may not receive communication services (IDEA, 2004). Such criteria are inappropriate when applied without considering an individual child's strengths and needs. Cognitive referencing is a particular concern because it assumes that a child's language and communication skills cannot improve beyond their cognitive ability. Notably, the research suggests that children with ID benefit from communication intervention even when there is no discrepancy between measures of language and cognition (Carr & Felice, 2000; Cole, Dale & Mills, 1990; Warren, Gazdag, Bambara, & Jones, 1994). Even adolescents and young adults with ID can benefit from communication intervention as their needs change with a focus more on developing functional communication to support peer interactions and success in a work setting (e.g., Cheslock, Barton-Hulsey, Romski, & Sevcik, 2008). Providers have a critical responsibility in ensuring their patients with ID receive those services necessary to maximize their independence and participation in their community.

Approaches to Intervention

Intervention for children with ID should minimize the potential debilitating effects of their disability while maximizing desirable outcomes (Wolery & Sainato, 1996). Primary healthcare providers have an important collaborative role in helping families and their children with ID achieve goals for health, safety, communication, and overall well-being. The SLP will be an important partner with the healthcare provider to ensure that the child with ID has an effective way to interact and master the environments, which may minimize or prevent future concerns and problems often associated with ID.

Based on initial and ongoing assessment data, children with ID have a unique profile related to their speech, language, hearing, and communication, cognitive level and behavior, and social-emotional status. Effective intervention capitalizes on a child's strengths across all areas of function to ensure an individualized and responsive intervention plan. The literature tells us that a child's level of functioning improves with personalize and sustained supports (AAIDD, 2013a, b). Primary healthcare providers must be aware of the individual profiles of their patients with ID and ensure that supports are in place to help the child achieve his/her full potential.

Some treatment principles should guide the dialogue with families and other providers who may be a part of the care team for a child with an ID. First, intervention should focus on interactions that children with ID encounter in their natural environments. Second, there should be sufficient opportunities for communication that incorporate language functions like requesting, greeting, and commenting with multiple communication partners. Finally, different communication forms and modalities (e.g., augmentative alternative communication (AAC) devices, pictures, signs, speech) should be available across home, school, recreational, and community contexts (Goldstein, 2006).

The targets for intervention, particularly communication intervention for children with ID, will depend on the assessment results as well as the child's age, etiology and severity of their condition, and overall communication and learning needs. Most often, intervention will consider enhancing a child's:

- Early communication skills including the ability to point, take turns, respond to joint attention bids, and initiate joint attention bids
- Social interaction and play with toys and other children
- Pragmatic skills or how they use language to communicate for a variety of purposes across context Speech production so their messages are intelligible
- Spoken and written language and literacy to support their school readiness
- Use of compensatory communication techniques such as assistive technology and AAC

Most intervention programs incorporate training for those who will be serving as communication partners for children with ID, and interprofessional collaboration is key to the child's communication success. For example, an SLP may work with primary healthcare providers to support their understanding of a child's expression of pain when the child is sick or hurt. Table 10.2 provides several examples of communication modalities and intervention approaches primary healthcare providers might hear about from the parents of a child with ID or see when the child makes an office visit.

Service delivery for children with ID can be home-based, pull-out with an identified therapist or clinician, classroom-based, and/or involve collaborative consultation. Pull-out approaches continue to predominant the delivery of related services, but it is a less appropriate method for supporting children with ID (Cirrin & Penner, 1995; Nelson, 1998). Early intervention is critical especially for those children with ID who are at high risk for communication disorders as intervention can influence development and cognitive and social outcomes (Guralnick, 2005; Ludlow & Allen, 1979; Mahoney & Perales, 2005; Ramey & Ramey, 1998). Setting is also a crucial ingredient for successful intervention. Implementation of intervention in everyday contexts or the child's natural environment is more likely to lead to generalized learning (Paul-Brown & Caperton, 2001).

Table 10.2 Examples of communication modalities and intervention approaches used for children with ID[a]

Communication modality/intervention approach	Description
Augmentative alternative communication (AAC)	Use of picture communication symbols, line drawings, Blissymbols, tangible objects, manual signs, gestures, finger spelling, speech-generating devices
Activity schedules/ visual supports	Display of objects, photographs, drawings, or written words that prompt a sequence of tasks/activities to completion, help focus attention to tasks, or facilitate transition from one task to another
Computer-based instruction	Use of computer technology (e.g., iPad) and/or software programs to teach communication and social skills
Video modeling	Use of video recordings that model desired behaviors which are then observed and imitated
Behavioral interventions	Implementation of different reinforcement, prompting, fading, and modeling to reduce behavior problems; review of what comes before (antecedents) and after (consequences) a behavior to make needed adjustments
Applied behavioral analysis (ABA)	Application of learning theory principles to elicit positive behavior change in behavior and build a variety of skills
Environmental arrangement	Arrangement of the environment to facilitate communication such as putting interesting materials in sight but out of reach, setting up choices, and creating unexpected situations
Functional communication training	Replacement of challenging behaviors with more appropriate communication alternatives
Incidental teaching	Elaboration on language initiated by a child while following the child's lead and reinforcing communication attempts in the natural environment
Milieu communication training	Use of systematic approaches to prompt children's ability to expand their communication functions and use increasingly complex language skills
Time delay	Use of a delay between an initial instruction and further prompting to increase a child's verbal production
Peer-mediated intervention	Incorporation of peers as communication partners in which they are taught strategies to facilitate play and social interactions in inclusive settings with children who have a variety of developmental disabilities

[a]See www.asha.org/practice-Portal/Clinical-Topics/Intellectual-Disability for additional information on these intervention approaches

Summary

Primary healthcare providers have a significant role in their support of families and children with ID. That support begins with assurance that the child has had a comprehensive assessment of his/her learning, adaptive functioning, and communication strengths and challenges. It also requires knowledge of associated health conditions so that the child receives appropriate and timely follow-up. Hearing and vision screening should be a routine part of the child's plan of care. Since there are a number of co-occurring conditions with ID, referral to a team with experience in differential diagnosis should be made. There are a number of approaches to supporting the success of children with ID, but early intervention is key, and eligibility for services must be understood. The SLP can support the primary healthcare provider by completing initial assessments of speech, language, hearing, and communication for children with ID and offer suggestions to support communication among the family, child, and provider. They can also explain processes for service eligibility and make recommendations for the most appropriate intervention approaches considering the child's individual needs and relative strengths, as well as the family's priority goals and desired outcomes.

References

American Association on Intellectual and Developmental Disabilities. (2013a). Definition of intellectual disability. Retrieved from www.aaidd.org

American Association on Intellectual and Developmental Disabilities. (2013b). The Supports Intensity Scale. Retrieved from www.aaidd.org

American Psychiatric Association. (2013). *Diagnostic and statistical manual of mental disorders* (5th ed.). Washington, DC: Author.

American Speech-Language Hearing Association. (2016, June). Childhood disability prevalence exceeds 1 in 7. *The ASHA Leader, 21*, 12.

Batshaw, M.L., Roizen, N., & Lotrecchiano, G.R. (2013). Children with disabilities, 7th edition. Baltimore: Brookes Publishing.

Brady, N. C., Bruce, S., Goldman, A., Erickson, K., Mineo, B., Ogletree, B. T., et al. (2016). Communication services and supports for individuals with severe disabilities: Guidance for assessment and intervention. *American Journal on Intellectual and Developmental Disabilities, 121*, 121–138.

Brault, M. W. (2012). *Americans with disabilities: 2010. Current Population Reports* (pp. P70–P131). Washington, DC: U.S. Census Bureau.

Carr, D., & Felice, D. (2000). Application of stimulus equivalence to language intervention with severe linguistic disabilities. *Journal of Intellectual and Developmental Disability, 25*, 181–205.

Cheslock, M., Barton-Hulsey, A., Romski, M. A., & Sevcik, R. A. (2008). Using a speech generating device to enhance communicative abilities and interactions for an adult with moderate intellectual disability: A case report. *Intellectual and Developmental Disabilities, 46*, 376–386.

Cirrin, F. M., & Penner, S. G. (1995). Classroom-based and consultative service delivery models for language intervention. In M. E. Fey, J. Windsor, & S. F. Warren (Eds.), *Language intervention: Preschool through the elementary years* (pp. 333–362). Baltimore, MD: Brookes.

Cole, K. N., Dale, P. S., & Mills, P. E. (1990). Defining language delay in young children by cognitive referencing: Are we saying more than we know? *Applied PsychoLinguistics, 11*, 291–302.

Developmental Disabilities Assistance and Bill of Rights Act (2000). Public Law106–402, 102(8). Retrieved from http://www.acl.gov/Programs/AIDD/DDA_BOR_ACT_2000/docs/dd_act.pdf

Gentile, J. P., Cowan, A. E., & Smith, A. B. (2015). Physical health of patients with intellectual disability. *Advances in Life Sciences and Health, 2*(1), 91–102.

Giangreco, M. F. (1990). Making related service decisions for students with severe disabilities: Roles, criteria, and authority. *Journal of the Association for Persons with Severe Handicaps, 15*(1), 22–31.

Goldstein, H. (2006). Clinical issues: Language intervention considerations for children with mental retardation and developmental disabilities. *Perspectives on Language Learning and Education, 13*(3), 21–26.

Guralnick, M. J. (2005). Early intervention for children with intellectual disabilities: Current knowledge and future prospects. *Journal of Applied Research in Intellectual Disabilities, 18*, 313–324.

Herer, G. R. (2012). Intellectual disabilities and hearing loss. *Communication Disorders Quarterly, 33*, 252–260.

Individuals with Disabilities Education Improvement Act. (2004). Public Law 108–446, 20 U.S.C. 1400 et seq.

Krahn, G. L., Hammond, L., & Turner, A. (2006). A cascade of disparities: Health and health care access for people with intellectual disabilities. *Mental Retardation and Developmental Disabilities Research Reviews, 12*, 70–82 Special Issue: Preventive Health and Individuals with Mental Retardation.

Ludlow, J. R., & Allen, L. M. (1979). The effect of early intervention and preschool stimulus on the development of the Downs syndrome child. *Journal of Intellectual Disability Research, 23*, 29–44.

Mahoney, G., & Perales, F. (2005). Relationship-focused early intervention with children with pervasive developmental disorders and other disabilities: A comparative study. *Journal of Developmental and Behavioral Pediatrics, 26*(2), 77–85.

Maulik, P. K., Mascarenhas, M. N., Mathers, C. D., Dua, T., & Saxena, S. (2011). Prevalence of intellectual disability: A meta-analysis of population-based studies. *Research in Developmental Disabilities, 32*, 419–436.

Maulik, P. K., Mascarenhas, M. N., Mathers, C. D., Dua, T., & Saxena, S. (2013). Corregendum to prevalence of intellectual disability: A meta-analysis of population-based studies [*Research in Developmental Disabilities 32*(2) (2011) 419–436]. *Research in Developmental Disabilities, 34*, 729.

McKenzie, K., Milton, M., Smith, G., & Ouellette-Kuntz, H. (2016). Systematic review of the prevalence and incidence of intellectual disabilities: Current trends and issues. *Current Development Disorders Report, 3*, 104–115.

National Joint Committee for the Communication Needs of Persons with Severe Disabilities. (1992). *Guidelines for meeting the communication needs of persons with severe disabilities* [Guidelines]. Available from www.asha.org/njc.

National Survey of Children with Special Health Care Needs. (2009/2010). Data query from the Child and Adolescent Health Measurement Initiative, Data Resource Center for Child and Adolescent Health website [NS-CSHCN 2009/10]. Retrieved from www.childhealthdata.org

Nelson, N. W. (1998). *Childhood language disorders in context: Infancy through adolescence*. Needham Heights, MA: Allyn & Bacon.

Oeseburg, B., Dijkstra, G. J., Groothoff, J. W., Reijneveld, S. I., & Jansen, D. E. M. C. (2011). Prevalence of chronic health conditions in children with intellectual disability: A systematic literature review. *Intellectual and Developmental Disabilities, 49*(2), 59–85.

Patja, K., Molska, P., & Iivanainen, M. (2001). Cause-specific mortality of people with intellectual disability in a population-based, 35-year follow-up study. *Journal of Intellectual Disability Research, 45*(1), 30–40.

Paul-Brown, D., & Caperton, C. (2001). Inclusive practices for preschool children with specific language impairment. In M. J. Guralnick (Ed.), *Early childhood inclusion: Focus on change* (pp. 433–463). Baltimore, MD: Brookes.

Ramey, C. T., & Ramey, S. L. (1998). Prevention of intellectual disabilities: Early interventions to improve cognitive development. *Preventive Medicine, 27*, 224–232.

Rimmer, J. H., Yamaki, K., Lowry, B. M. D., Wang, E., & Vogel, L. C. (2010). Obesity and obesity-related secondary conditions in adolescents with intellectual/developmental disabilities. *Journal of Intellectual Disability Research, 54*, 787–794.

Schalock, R. L., Luckasson, R. A., & Shorgren, K. A. (2007). The renaming of *Mental Retardation*: Understanding the change to the term intellectual disability. *Intellectual and Developmental Disabilities, 45*, 116–124.

Schieve, L. A., Gonzalez, V., Boulet, S. L., Visser, S. N., Rice, C. E., Braun, K. V. N., & Boyle, C. A. (2012). Concurrent medical conditions and health care use and needs among children with learning and behavioral developmental disabilities, National Health Interview Survey, 2006-2010. *Research in Developmental Disabilities, 33*, 467–476.

Sparrow, S., Cicchetti, D. V., & Balla, D. A. (2005). *Vineland adaptive behavior scales* (2nd ed.). Circle Pines, MN: American Guidance Services.

Sullivan, W. F., Berg, J. M., Bradley, E., Cheetham, T., Denton, R., Heng, J., et al. (2011). Primary care of adults with developmental disabilities Canadian consensus guidelines. *Canadian Family Physician, 57*, 541–553.

U. S. Department of Education. (2015). EDFacts Data Warehouse (EDW): IDEA Part B Child Count and Educational Environments Collection, 2014–15. Data extracted as of July 2, 2015 from file specifications 002 and 089.

van Schrojenstein Lantman-de Valk, H. M. J., & Noonan Walsh, P. (2008). Managing health problems in people with intellectual disabilities. *British Medical Journal, 337*, 1408–1412.

Warburg, M. (2001). Visual impairment in adult people with intellectual disability: Literature review. *Journal of Intellectual Disability Research, 45*, 424–438.

Warren, S. F., Gazdag, G., Bambara, L., & Jones, H. (1994). Changes in the generativity and use of sematic relationships concurrent with milieu language intervention. *Journal of Speech and Hearing Research, 37*, 924–934.

Wolery, M., & Sainato, D. (1996). General curriculum and intervention strategies. In S. Odom & M. McLean (Eds.), *Early intervention/early childhood special education: Recommended practices* (pp. 125–158). PRO-ED: Austin, TX.

World Health Organization. (2001). *ICF: International classification of functioning, disability and health*. Geneva, Switzerland: Author.

World Health Organization. (2007). *ICF-CY: International classification of functioning, disability and health: Children & youth version*. Geneva, Switzerland: Author.

Chapter 11
Children with Attention-Deficit/Hyperactivity Disorder

Introduction

Many children have some inattention or unfocused motor activity and impulsivity, but for children with attention-deficit/hyperactivity disorder (ADHD), this inattention, overactivity, and impulsivity appear to be more severe, occur more frequently, and typically compromise a child's ability to function at home and school. ADHD is considered a brain disorder characterized by inattention and/or hyperactivity and impulsivity. More specifically, inattention suggests a child might wander off task displaying difficulty with sustained focus and persistence, while hyperactivity suggests a child is in constant motion particularly in situations where such activity is inappropriate with a tendency to fidget and talk excessively. A child who is impulsive usually requires immediate rewards or gratification and acts before thinking which puts the child at risk for harm. ADHD is most commonly diagnosed in school-age children, affecting approximately 5 to 7% of the student population, and is a chronic disorder impacting an individual throughout life although symptom severity tends to decrease with age (Willcutt, 2012).

The symptoms characterizing ADHD can impact the communication skills of children which is the focus of this chapter. In fact, some children with ADHD symptoms may have an undiagnosed language deficit or a co-occurring communication disorder that complicates their condition. In this chapter, ADHD will be defined, highlighting the criteria for diagnosis. Then the prevalence, possible causes, and cultural differences in identifying the disorder will be discussed. Those symptoms that likely impact a child's ability to communicate and socially interact including the role of attention in the development of language will be emphasized, and issues of comorbidity will be presented. Finally, the importance of a comprehensive approach to assessment and intervention will be discussed.

P. A. Prelock, T. L. Hutchins, *Clinical Guide to Assessment and Treatment of Communication Disorders*, Best Practices in Child and Adolescent Behavioral Health Care, https://doi.org/10.1007/978-3-319-93203-3_11

Diagnosis and Prevalence of ADHD

The updated description for ADHD in the DSM-5 (APA, 2013) focuses on increasing the utility of the criteria to diagnose ADHD in adults and recognizes that although ADHD is a condition typically diagnosed in childhood, it likely extends through adulthood. The criteria for diagnosis did not change, but additional examples are provided to illustrate the kinds of behaviors children, adolescents, and adults must display. The number of symptoms required for a diagnosis remained at six for children and adolescents but dropped to five for adults as this number was sufficient for a reliable diagnosis. There was a change in age of onset, as the literature suggested symptoms should be present prior to 12 instead of 7 years. The exclusion criterion for children with ASD was eliminated in the DSM-5, recognizing both ASD and ADHD can co-occur. Behaviors must be persistent for 6 months, evident in at least two settings, and impact social, occupational, or educational function. The diagnostic criteria for ADHD inattentive and impulsive types are listed below:

ADHD Inattentive Type

- Failure to give close attention to details
- Difficulty in attention in daily tasks or play
- Difficulty in listening when spoken to
- Lack of follow through to finish activities
- Difficulty in organizing tasks
- Avoidance or dislike of sustained mental effort tasks
- Easily losing tools required for completion of tasks
- Easily distractible or forgetful

ADHD Impulsive Type

- Fidgets hands or feet or squirms when sitting
- Leaves his or her seat in class often when seating is expected
- Runs about or climbs often when these behaviors are not appropriate for the time and setting
- Has difficulty when playing or when trying to engage in leisure activities.
- Acts as if "driven by a motor"
- Talks excessively
- Blurts out answers before a question has been completed
- Has difficulty waiting for his or her turn or interrupts others often

Notably, ADHD can occur as a combined type with a child exhibiting both inattention and impulsivity.

Prevalence and Possible Causes

Approximately 11% of US children (or 6.4 million) have received a diagnosis of ADHD (Visser et al., 2014) with a steady increase in diagnosis noted from 1997 to 2006 (Pastor & Reuben, 2008). Notably, a 42% increase in diagnosis in 8 years from

2003–2004 to 2011–2012 raised questions regarding the validity of the diagnosis in the USA (Walkup, Stossel, & Rendleman, 2014). This is important as it suggests a need to more carefully attend to the symptoms and provide adequate differential diagnosis so that children with other possible difficulties (e.g., learning disorders, communication disorders) are appropriately identified. Visser et al. (2015) examined the experiences of US children diagnosed with ADHD as of 2011–2012 with data drawn from the 2014 National Survey of the Diagnosis and Treatment of ADHD and Tourette syndrome. Median age of diagnosis was 7 years although one third of the children were diagnosed prior to age 6. Those making the diagnosis ranged from primary healthcare providers to specialists in the diagnosis of childhood disorders such as psychologists, neurologists, and psychiatrists. Pediatricians, however, were the most likely to make the initial diagnosis. At least two thirds of the time families raised the initial concerns regarding their child's ability to attend, while school personnel raised concerns one third of the time.

Gender differences in diagnosis exist with a ratio ranging from 2:1 to 10:1 boys to girls in clinic samples and 2.5:1 to 5.1:1 boys to girls in epidemiological studies (Arnold, 1996). Notably, since the diagnostic criteria focus on acting out behavior, it seems likely that boys have an increased risk of receiving a diagnosis. It may be that girls have to exhibit greater symptom severity to be identified (Abikoff et al., 2002; Arnold et al., 1997; Gaub & Carlson, 1997; Gershon, 2002). Generally, the cause of ADHD is unknown although genetics appears to play a role and familial history reveals behaviors associated with ADHD. In fact, recent research indicates that nearly half of parents of children with ADHD also have the condition which has implications for the approach to parent training and the parents' educational style (Starck, Grunwald, & Schlarb, 2016). There is also evidence of brain abnormalities in children with ADHD (Valera & Seidman, 2006). The evidence we do have would suggest ADHD is real and not caused by watching too much TV or children eating sugary snacks as has been speculated in the popular press.

Cultural Considerations

Although ADHD may be perceived differently in different cultural contexts, it occurs across cultural systems. That is, the interpretation of symptom expression for ADHD is likely to be influenced by a child's culture, but the core features of ADHD seem to be equivalent across cultures. Most research has been done in the USA regarding symptom expression, but there are some interesting findings regarding the likely diagnostic outcomes in different cultures. For example, using the norms for the Child Behavior Checklist, 45% of children from Puerto Rico would be identified with ADHD, yet in Puerto Rico, high activity levels are expected in children – they move around and interrupt when they have something to say (Achenbach et al., 1990; Bauermeister, 1995; Bird, et al., 1988). Using an ADHD rating scale (based on the DSM-IV criteria), teachers rated children who were African American higher than students who were Caucasian on all symptoms; twice the number scored as positive for ADHD (Reid et al., 1998). Chinese, Japanese, Indonesian, and American professionals rated videos of children using the DSM criteria for ADHD; Chinese and Indonesian professionals had higher ratings than did American and Japanese professionals with the former groups seeming less tolerant of increased activity level and decreased attention in children (Mann et al., 1992; Mueller et al., 1995). Asian teachers rated students who were Asian more active than English teachers who rated students who were Caucasian using an actometer (machine that measures movement), yet there was no significant difference in the actual movement that occurred (Sonuga-Barke, Minocha, Taylor, & Sandberg, 1993).

Research has also occurred with Native and non-Native US children (Beiser, Dion, & Gotowiec 2000) using data from parents and teachers participating in a large-scale study of mental health and academic achievement. Results of parent and teacher reports indicated that attention deficit and hyperactivity-impulsivity are separable and distinct, yet no culture-bound symptoms were revealed in this study.

Thus, it seems that there are culture-specific norms and values for children's behavior that influence adults' conceptions of the presence of ADHD. At the same time, there is an undercurrent of real and invariant cognitive and behavioral ADHD symptoms that exist across cultures although these symptoms may be present with different degrees of severity. It is important, then, that primary healthcare providers are aware of the influence of culture and expectations for behavior based on a child's perceived activity level.

Role of Attention in Language and Communication

A child's ability to attend to the perceptual attributes of objects and actions provides input important for classifying and categorizing information, and children more easily respond to input that changes and is louder and brighter (e.g., toys changing colors with bright lights and musical sounds or activities that involve movements and exaggerated sounds). Objects and activities sharing these characteristics may influence early language learning. Children who are distractible and inattentive, however, are likely to miss out on important information, particularly if they only attend to the loudest things they hear, to the brightest things they see, or in settings where stimuli change frequently. Auditory attention requires a purposeful focus on relevant versus irrelevant acoustic information and is critical to learning as a child's capacity to decode all incoming signals is likely compromised if they have a language impairment (which may ultimately lead to greater inattention).

The inattention, hyperactivity, and/or impulsivity of a child with ADHD can negatively impact the child's ability to understand what is being said (receptive language), to produce a relevant response (expressive language), and to use language appropriately in social contexts (pragmatic language). Table 11.1 describes the likely impact on language function for several of the criteria characterizing children with ADHD. It is important that primary healthcare providers recognize the likely impact of ADHD on all aspects of child's functioning, particularly communication, as this has far-reaching implications for the child's success at home, in school, in the community, and with friends.

Table 11.1 Likely impact of ADHD on children's receptive, expressive, and pragmatic language function

Selected ADHD criteria	Likely impact on receptive language	Likely impact on expressive language	Likely impact on pragmatic language
Failure to give close attention to details	May miss important information to support comprehension across contexts	May repeat questions to get information already stated or offer inaccurate or incomplete information	May miss verbal and nonverbal cues regarding the intention, desire, and perspective of a speaker
Difficulty in attention in daily tasks or play	May misunderstand important information during lengthy reading tasks	May make repeated mistakes in written language tasks	May influence ability to initiate and sustain play with peers and ultimately establish friendships
Difficulty in listening when spoken to	May misinterpret instructions or comments	May respond without clear understanding of a previous question or comment	May risk misunderstanding in conversations with peers and adults
Difficulty in organizing tasks	May risk ability to study and prepare for tests or assignments	May jeopardize ability to formulate a narrative or expository essay or report	May miss appointments or planned activities with friends
Avoidance or dislike of sustained mental effort tasks	May impair ability to comprehend a lengthy and complex reading assignment	May impact ability to complete complex written tasks	May compromise ability to support a friend in a difficult situation
Easily distractible or forgetful	May impact ability to monitor speech or language errors in oral or written communication	May influence ability to retrieve and produce expected responses to tests or assignments	May jeopardize sustained interactions with peers or maintaining conversations
Has difficulty waiting for his or her turn or interrupts others	May lack comprehension monitoring necessary to complete work in cooperative groups	May risk accuracy in formulating responses to questions or comments	May compromise peer interactions in cooperative and pretend play
Blurts out answers before a question has been completed	May fail to fully understand what is being asked	May impact accuracy in responding to questions asked	May inhibit reciprocal exchanges in conversations
Talks excessively	May fail to monitor a listener's comprehension and interest	May produce unnecessary or irrelevant comments and questions	May jeopardize opportunities for successful conversations with peers and adults

As summarized in Table 11.1, pragmatic language problems are common in children with ADHD (Kim & Kaiser, 2000; Westby & Cutler, 1994). Children with ADHD have difficulty using effective communication skills in specific educational and social situations. For example, conversational skills are compromised because of difficulties taking turns, the tendency to interrupt, and the propensity to talk excessively. Children with ADHD are likely to initiate conversational exchanges at inappropriate times, switch topics without warning, present disconnected thoughts, use poor eye contact, or have difficulty adapting their message to the listener (Bruce, Thernlund, & Nettelbladt 2006; Geurts et al., 2004). Children with ADHD also exhibit less accurate interpretations of referential statements, which likely contribute to their challenges in conversations and interpersonal relationships as they fail to understand the perspective of the speaker (Nilsen, Mangal, & MacDonald, 2013). It appears that children with ADHD have more performance than knowledge deficits in pragmatic language. At the same time, they also appear to have greater difficulty in the area of expressive speech and language as revealed in impaired sentence imitation, word articulation, and overall performance on standard measures of language (Kim & Kaiser, 2000). In community samples of children without ADHD, higher levels of inattention and hyperactivity- impulsivity are associated with greater pragmatic language deficits (Bignell & Cain, 2007; Ketelaars, Cuperus, Jansonius, & Verhoeven, 2010; Leonard, Milich, & Lorch, 2011), while in children with ADHD, pragmatic language skills are poor compared to typically developing children and rival the pragmatic deficits observed in autism spectrum disorder (Bishop & Baird; 2001; Bruce et al., 2006; Geurts & Embrechts, 2008; Guerts et al., 2004; Helland, Biringer, Helland, & Heimann, 2012; Helland & Heimann, 2007).

Related social skill challenges that characterize the behavior of children with ADHD include poor self-talk to monitor and organize their interpersonal behavior; failure to read verbal, nonverbal, and environmental cues; and an aggressive interaction style that is seen as disruptive and intrusive by their peers often causing rejection (Kim & Kaiser, 2000). In addition, children with ADHD often fail to attend to the requests or initiations of the peers and are unable to adjust their interaction style to different situations with a variety of communication partners.

Children with ADHD also demonstrate meta-cognitive language problems that involve challenges organizing, planning, monitoring, and evaluating their behavior including difficulty integrating multiple pieces of information. In narrative language tasks, for example, they use fewer causal connections in stories, have difficulty with goal establishment, and make less frequent mention of initiating events than children without ADHD (Flory et al., 2006). They also exhibit problems with causal story structures to guide their comprehension and later recall. Children with ADHD use more ambiguous references, include more extraneous information in their narratives, and have less success answering inferential questions than children without ADHD (Flory et al., 2006; Lorch et al., 1999; McInnes, Humphries, Hogg- Johnson & Tannock, 2003; Renz et al., 2003).

Written language difficulties in ADHD have also been reported in the literature. Children with ADHD score lower than their peers on measures of written language adequacy, structure, grammar, and vocabulary (Re et al., 2007). They also produce shorter texts and make more errors than matched controls (Re et al., 2007). Written language difficulties are likely due to the planning and organizational challenges of children with ADHD.

There is some evidence of theory of mind challenges, particularly in the area of emotion recognition that appear to characterize the responses of school-age children with ADHD. They appear to be less accurate than their typical peers in identifying the emotions of happiness, sadness, anger, and fear in pictures and in the tone of voice of an adult reading a sentence (Cadesky, Mota, & Schachar, 2000). Children with ADHD were also less accurate in their ability to identify anger and sadness when shown photographs depicting joy, anger, disgust, and sadness in varying intensities (Pelc, Kornreich, Foisy, & Dan, 2006). These challenges in emotion recognition are important as there appears to be a correlation between interpersonal problems and impairment in decoding emotional facial expressions.

Some relationships have been reported between language and ADHD-like behaviors in preschool children (Armstrong & Nettleton, 2004) that are important to recognize and address. A young child's inattention or impulsivity can disrupt joint attention activities which can impact the effectiveness of parental language models. Joint attention is a critical skill to the early theory of mind and play development. A mother's response to her young child's ADHD behavior may also disrupt language learning (i.e., problematic behaviors may lead to more directive vs. facilitative interaction styles) and can affect parental use of scaffolding strategies important to language learning (Camarata & Gibson, 1999). The impact of attention on early language development is important as diminished language skills heighten the likelihood of behavioral problems frequently associated with ADHD.

Issues of Comorbidity

Knowing there are implications of ADHD on a child's ability to understand, express, and use his or her communication in meaningful learning and social contexts, it is important to recognize issues of comorbidity. This also raises the importance of differential diagnosis and a comprehensive assessment of a child's individual strengths, challenges, and needs. Fletcher et al. (2000) have discussed the relationships among learning disability, language disorder, and ADHD. They suggest that both a learning disability and language disorder represent a disorder of cognition, while ADHD is a behavioral disorder with implications for cognitive function. Yet, all three seem to originate from brain differences and impact cognition. As was described in Chap. 7, a learning disability is manifested in academic problems involving the ability to listen, think, talk, read, write, spell, and do math, while a language disorder (see Chap. 6) is an impairment in comprehension and/or the use of spoken, written, or other symbol system that involves the form, content, and function of language. In contrast, ADHD does not have widely accepted performance-based indicators and instead represents a deficit in rule-governed behavior that relates to language challenges and involves cognitive function. Children with inattention appear to be lethargic, daydreamers, distractible, and unfocused, while those with impulsivity have deficits in response to inhibition which impacts cognitive functions like working memory, self-regulation, internalization of speech, and reconstruction or the creation of alternative response strategies to feedback (Fletcher, Aram, Shaywitz, & Shaywitz, 2000).

ADHD has been one of the most frequently reported co-occurring neurodevelopmental disorders in study samples of children with language impairments (LI) (Beitchman, Hood, & Inglis, 1990; Benasich, Curtiss, & Tallal, 1993; Kim & Kaiser, 2000; Lindsay, Dockrell, & Strand, 2007; Love & Thompson, 1988; St. Clair, Pickles, Durkin, & Conti-Ramsden, 2011; Trautman, Giddan, & Jurs, 1990; Willinger et al., 2003). Although the literature provides some discrepant findings with the extent to which co-occurrence rates have exceeded expectations based on general population estimates, it remains an important finding (Lindsay & Dockrell, 2008; Redmond & Rice, 2002; Rescorla, Ross, & McClure, 2007; Whitehouse, Robinson, & Zubrick, 2011).With the overlap of characteristics in both the criteria for ADHD and language disorders, there are some challenges in differential diagnosis, and often assessment tools to assess language also identify weaknesses in attention and task completion (Tetnowski, 2004). On language measures, however, children with ADHD alone appear to understand and produce a greater number of words and a greater number of different words than children with language impairment, and their mean length of utterance is longer than that of children with language disorders (Tetnowski, 2004). Children with both ADHD and language-based learning disabilities (LLD), however, have significantly more problems formulating grammatically correct sentences and planning, organizing, and sequencing oral, written, and behavioral responses than their peers or children with ADHD or LLD alone (Javorsky, 1996). Assessments of pragmatic language (e.g., figurative language, inferencing, cohesion in narratives and conversation) in children with co-occurring language impairment and ADHD suggest that even mild differences in figurative language knowledge contributes to social problem-solving deficits in adolescents with psychopathologies (Im-bolter, Cohen, & Farnia, 2013).

There are instances when children with a specific learning disability may appear to be inattentive as a result of "frustration, lack of interest, or limited ability. However, inattention in individuals with a specific learning disorder who do not have ADHD is not impairing outside of academic work" (APA, 2013, p. 64). This would be a differentiating characteristic of children with ADHD vs. a learning disability. There are times, though, when ADHD and a learning disability co-occur. In adolescents, there are other implications for psychosocial status with the co-occurrence of a learning disability and ADHD. Learning disabilities (LD) appear to serve as a risk factor for more negative outcomes in adolescents with ADHD (McNamara, Willoughby, & Chalmers, & YLC-CURA, 2005). McNamara et al. (2005) found that adolescents with comorbid LD/ADHD had poorer maternal relationships than adolescents with LD alone or those who were typically developing and more instances of being shoved, sworn at, called names, teased, and ridiculed. Recognizing the additive effects of LD with ADHD suggests that primary healthcare providers, families, and school teams need to put protective factors in place to act as buffers against the presence of LD.

Reading disabilities and ADHD are also frequently reported as co-occurring in school-age children (Pisecco, Baker, Silva, & Brooke, 2001). Reading challenges include failure to monitor comprehension, failure to understand main ideas and difficulty inferencing, and failure to use language to regulate behavior and plan (McInnes, et al., 2003). Generally, it seems that ADHD and reading problems are at least partially distinct but co-occur.

Assessment Considerations

Behavior rating scales and checklists are most often used to determine a diagnosis of ADHD. It is important to have such scales or checklists completed by both parents and teachers to document the occurrence of suspected attention challenges across at least two settings. Notably, about 68% of children suspected of having an ADHD also receive a neuropsychological assessment, although those diagnosed at younger ages are more likely to receive this testing than those diagnosed after 6 years of age. Approximately 30% of children may also receive neuroimaging or laboratory tests.

Child psychiatrists, developmental pediatricians, or other trained and experienced healthcare professionals (e.g., psychologists) with expertise in the diagnosis of ADHD should be those responsible for making a diagnosis. The diagnosis should be made on the basis of a full clinical and psychosocial assessment of the child including information gathered from discussions about the child's behavior and symptoms in the different settings and different aspects of the child's life (American Academy of Pediatrics (AAP), 2011). This assessment should include a full developmental and psychiatric history and observer reports of the child's behavior. A diagnosis should never be made on the basis of a rating scale or observational data alone (AAP, 2011).

Co-occurring ADHD and communication disorders are an assessment challenge for school-based practitioners who must determine the source of a child's academic and social difficulties as either language-based, attention-based, or a combination of both. Considering the frequency with which language disorders and other learning disorders co-occur with ADHD, an assessment of a child's language and learning status is critical as problems in these areas could be misconstrued as an ADHD without thoughtful differential diagnosis. In addition, since language and learning disorders often co-occur with ADHD, it is important to assess these aspects of a child's functioning to identify other potential risk factors and needs for the child.

A speech-language pathologist (SLP) can be particularly helpful in providing the needed language and social pragmatic assessments for children with or suspected of an ADHD. The SLP is able to observe interactions and conversations with peers and teachers in both classroom and formal testing situations. SLPs also interview caregivers about their child's speech and language development and interview the child to assess his or her self-awareness of challenge areas. In addition to the typical assessment of speech, fluency, language comprehension, and language production, SLPs have expertise in evaluating a child's ability to tell or retell a story; to plan, organize, and attend to details in both oral and written language; and to recognize and discuss different perspectives of characters in stories.

Further, SLPs can assess a child's social communication skills or their pragmatic language function – how they use language in various social contexts. They may use the *Children's Communication Checklist-2* (Bishop, 2003) to examine pragmatics in children 4 to 16 years or evaluate conversational or narrative discourse using a variety language and narrative analysis methods (Fey, 1991; Hedberg & Westby, 1993; Hughes, McGillivray & Schmidek, 1997; Retherford, 2000). They may also use the *Social Skills Rating Scale* (Gresham & Elliot, 1990) which includes parent, teacher, and self-report and is appropriate for assessing a child's social skills, problem behaviors, and the impact on academic performance from preschool through high school.

Intervention Considerations

Behavioral approaches (AAP, 2001, 2011; Barkley, 1998; Pelham, Wheeler, & Chronis, 1998; US DOE, 2003) are frequently used to modify the physical and social environment of children with ADHD to increase their appropriate behavior and alter their undesired behavior. Table 11.2 outlines key behavioral strategies that are recommended for both parents and teachers. These approaches include direct teaching and reinforcement for positive behaviors and consequences for inappropriate behaviors.

Unfortunately, behavioral approaches have had mixed results. Programs that are systematic with contingency management in specialized classrooms and summer camps with well-trained individuals are highly effective (Abramowitz, Eckstrand, O'Leary, & Dulcan, 1992; Carlson, Pelham, Milich, & Dixon, 1992; Pelham & Hoza, 1996). Parent training in behavior therapy and classroom behavior interventions also indicate positive change in the behavior of children with ADHD (Pelham, et al., 1998). Because many interventions are associated with medications, analysis of effectiveness of behavioral treatments alone is difficult as is an assessment of treatment maintenance (AAP, 2001; Rapport, Stoner, & Jones, 1986). Some research indicates that behavioral interventions are not as effective as psychostimulant treatment (Jadad, Boyle & Cunningham, 1999; Pelham et al., 1998). It is clear that behavioral interventions must be implemented and maintained to be effective (AAP, 2001, 2011).

Table 11.2 Behavioral strategies to support desired behaviors in children with ADHD

Behavioral strategy	Description
Behavioral training for parents and teachers	Learn child behavior management strategies
Systematic program of contingency management	Positive reinforcement, time-out, response cost, token economy
Clinical behavioral therapy	Training in problem-solving and social skills
Cognitive behavioral treatment	Self-monitoring, verbal self-instruction, self-reinforcement

Pharmacological approaches are also common with some controversy. Stimulants are frequently used with the expectation that children will be better able to attend to critical aspects of their environment, and this result is often seen in 75% or more of children who are taking the medication (NIMH, 2000). A multimodal treatment study comparing the use of medication alone to medication plus behavioral intervention indicated that the use of medication was almost as effective medication and behavioral interventions (Edwards, 2002; Jensen, 2001; MTA Cooperative group, 1999a, 1999b). At the moment, however, the quality of the available evidence suggests we cannot say for sure whether taking methylphenidate, for example, will improve the lives of children and adolescents with ADHD (Storebo et al., 2015). Methylphenidate, the most frequently used stimulant medication, is associated with a number of nonserious adverse events such as problems with sleeping and decreased appetite. Although the evidence does not suggest an increased risk of serious adverse events, trials with longer follow-up are needed to better assess the risk of serious adverse events in children who take methylphenidate over a long period of time (Storebo et al., 2015). Further, there remain limitations in medication effectiveness because of persistent problems with medication compliance and the lack of generalized positive effects to broader areas of life functioning including academic achievement, executive function, motivation, and self-regulation.

There are also self-regulation approaches that can be incorporated into the intervention plan for a child with ADHD (Lienemann & Reid, 2008; Reid, Trout, & Schartz, 2005). These include a number of strategies that students are taught to use to manage, monitor, record, and/or assess their behavior and academic performance (Mace, Belfiore, & Hutchinson, 2001). Table 11.3 presents a summary of these self-regulatory approaches which are effective in increasing children's on-task behaviors and academic productivity and accuracy as well as decreasing inappropriate or disruptive behaviors (Reid et al., 2005).

Interventions for children with ADHD and language disorders must incorporate language intervention if students are to understand the structure and rules of discourse and conversation. There are several strategies SLPs may incorporate in an intervention plan for children with ADHD who also exhibit language problems.

Table 11.3 Self-regulation approaches for supporting children with ADHD

Self-regulation strategy	Description
Self-monitoring	Observe one's behavior (e.g., performance or attention) through self-recording and graphing a target response
Self-monitoring + reinforcement	Implement the self-monitoring approach described above and increase the salience and importance by an external agent rewarding positive changes in target behaviors
Self-reinforcement	Reward own behavior when a predetermined performance standard is met
Self-management or self-evaluation	Monitor, rate, and compare an aspect of behavior with an external standard or criteria; self-assess and self-record at set intervals; reinforce if recordings are similar to an external observer

Eliminating environmental distractions, redirecting the child, and providing verbal, visual, and tactile feedback can facilitate a child's attention recall. The use of whole-body activities such as identifying the parts of the body used to listen, highlighting what attending behaviors look like, and differentiating between "hearing" and "listening" can also facilitate a child's understanding of how to listen in academic and social situations. There is some research that suggests children with language and attention difficulties may benefit from prior listening experiences, and practicing language processing similar to expository text may facilitate a children's focus when they are exposed to linguistic distractions (Dalebout, Nelson, Hletko, & Frentheway, 1991). Other strategies might include requiring children to repeat instructions, record instructions so they can listen to them again, and use simple, single directions (Heyer, 1995).

Since the classroom is often an environment with competing noises and listening challenges for children with language and attention problems, sound field amplification has been used to improve classroom listening for children in the elementary grades (Elliot et al., 1989; Flexer, Wray, & Ireland, 1989). Other whole language classroom strategies that are recommended for children with language and attention difficulties include giving learning choices, encouraging creative thinking and mobility in the classroom, organizing the environment for learning, and building on strengths (Weaver, 1993). Using thematic-based learning is also facilitative for children with language and attention problems as it creates a predictable structure for the child to follow, can build on familiar scripts, and supports collaborative learning activities.

For younger children with attention problems and language challenges, there are a number of treatment strategies that might be considered. These include (Giddan & Milling, 2000; McGoey, Eckert, & DuPaul, 2002; Tetter, 1998):

- Providing a consistent program structure and routine
- Using visual schedules and other organizing aids
- Giving clear, simple, and individual instructions
- Allowing motor activities as a break between structured activities
- Providing consistent, strong, and immediate feedback
- Implementing positive reinforcement for desired behavior
- Integrating a behavior management program across settings

Speech and language intervention for children with ADHD is always individualized and will likely focus on teaching communication in specific social situations. If medication is prescribed, the SLP collaborates with other educational professionals to observe the child's behavior prior to and following medication use. The SLP will communicate with the family and physician regarding any observed changes. The SLP also works with the teacher to change the classroom environment as needed.

Summary

Primary healthcare providers have an important role in understanding the complexities of diagnosing children with ADHD, including recognizing possible comorbidities and the impact of language impairments or learning disorders on a child's ability to attend as well as the risk children with ADHD have for communication and academic difficulties. Assessment should be comprehensive and include not only behavior rating scales but a full battery of neuropsychological and language testing. A referral to an SLP is critical for children suspected of having an ADHD because of their risk for pragmatic language deficits and social interaction challenges. It is also important to rule out a language disorder as a possible reason for observed challenges in attending. There are several approaches to intervention with a combination of behavioral and pharmacological strategies used most often. Importantly, though, the behavioral interventions must be maintained to achieve positive long-term outcomes, and the use of self-regulatory strategies has value in empowering children with ADHD to self-manage their behavior. SLPs incorporate several strategies in their work with children with ADHD and language deficits including ways to increase the salience of the auditory signal, streamline instructions given, and provide visual supports and instructional aides to facilitate a child's ability to listen and comprehend. Routines, schedules, organizing everyday items and activities, instructional clarity and consistency, and rewards for appropriate behaviors are all strategies that can support the daily success of a child with ADHD (retrieved on October 20, 2016 at www.nimh.nih.gov/health/topics/attention-deficit-hyperactivity-disorder).

References

Abikoff, H. B., Jensen, P. S., Eugene, L. L., Hoza, B., Hetchman, L., Pollack, S., et al. (2002). Observed classroom behavior of children with ADHD: Relationships to gender and comorbidity. *Journal of Abnormal Child Psychology, 30*(4), 349–359.

Abramowitz, A. J., Eckstrand, D., O'Leary, S. G., & Dulcan, M. K. (1992). ADHD children's responses to stimulant medication and two intensities of a behavioral intervention. *Behavior Modification, 16*, 193–203.

Achenbach, T., Bird, H. R., Canino, G., Phares, V., Gould, M. S., & Rubio-Stipec, M. (1990). Epidemiological comparisons of Puerto Rican and U.S. mainland children: Parent and teacher self-report. *Journal of the American Academy of Child & Adolescent Psychiatry, 29*, 84–93.

American Academy of Pediatrics. (2001). Clinical practice guideline: Treatment of the school-aged child with attention deficit/hyperactivity disorder. *Pediatrics, 108*, 1033–1044.

American Academy of Pediatrics. (2011). ADHD: Clinical practice guideline for the diagnosis, evaluation and treatment of ADHD in children and adolescents. *Pediatrics, 128*(5), 1007–1022.

American Psychiatric Association. (2013). *Diagnostic and statistical manual of mental disorders, DSM-5* (5th ed.). Washington, DC: APA.

Armstrong, M. B., & Nettleton, S. K. (2004). ADHD and preschool children. *Seminars in Speech & Language, 25*(3), 225–232.

Arnold, L. S. (1996). Sex differences in ADHD: Conference summary. *Journal of Abnormal Psychology, 24*, 555–569.

Arnold, L. S., Abikoff, H. B., Cantwell, D. P., Conners, C. K., Elliott, G. R., Greenhill, L. L., et al. (1997). NIMH collaborative multimodal treatment study of children with ADHD (MTA): Design challenges and choices. *Archives of General Psychiatry, 54*, 865–870.

Barkley, R. A. (1998). *Handbook of attention deficit hyperactivity disorder* (2nd ed.). New York: Guilford Press.

Bauermeister, J. J. (1995). Teacher rating scales for the assessment of ADDD and ADHD in Hispanic (Puerto Rican) children. *The ADHD Report, 3*, 9–10.

Benasich, A., Curtiss, S., & Tallal, P. (1993). Language, learning, and behavioral disturbance in childhood: A longitudinal perspective. *Journal of the American Academy of Child and Adolescent Psychiatry, 32*, 585–594.

Beiser, M., Dion, R., & Gotowiec, A. (2000). The structure of attention-deficit and hyperactivity symptoms among native and non-native elementary school children. *Journal of Abnormal Child Psychology, 28*(5), 425–437.

Beitchman, J., Hood, J., & Inglis, A. (1990). Psychiatric risk in children with speech and language disorders. *Journal of Abnormal Child Psychology, 18*(3), 283–296.

Bignell, S., & Cain, K. (2007). Pragmatic aspects of communication and language comprehension in groups of children differentiated by teacher ratings of hyperactivity and inattention. *British Journal of Developmental Psychology, 25*, 499–512.

Bird, H., Canino, G., Rubio-Stipec, M., Gould, M. S., Ribera, J., Sesman, M., et al. (1988). Estimates of the prevalence of childhood maladjustment in a community survey in Puerto Rico. *Archives of General Psychiatry, 45*, 1120–1126.

Bishop, D. V. M. (2003). *The Children's Communication Checklist, CCC-2* (2nd ed.). London: Psychological Corp.

Bishop, D., & Baird, G. (2001). Parent and teacher report of pragmatic aspects of communication: Use of the Children's Communication Checklist in a clinical setting. *Developmental Medicine & Child Neurology, 43*, 809–819.

Bruce, B., Thernlund, G., & Nettelbladt, U. (2006). ADHD and language impairment: A study of the parent questionnaire FTF (Five to Fifteen). *European Child and Adolescent Psychiatry, 15*, 52–60.

Cadesky, E.B., Mota, V.L., & Schachar, R.J., (2000). Beyond words: How do children with ADHD and/or conduct problems process nonverbal information about affect? *Journal of American Academy of Child and Adolescent Psychiatry, 39*, 1160–1167.

Camarata, S., & Gibson, T. (1999). Pragmatic language deficits in ADHD. *Mental Retardation and Developmental Disabilities, 5*, 207–214.

Carlson, C. L., Pelham Jr., W. E., Milich, R., & Dixon, J. (1992). Single and combined effects of methylphenidate and behavior therapy on the classroom performance of children with attention-deficit hyperactivity disorder. *Journal of Abnormal Child Psychology, 20*, 213–232.

Geurts, H., & Embrechts, M. (2008). Language Profiles in ASD, SLI, and ADHD. *Journal of Autism and Developmental Disorders, 38*, 1931–1943.

Geurts, H., Verte, S., Oosterlaan, J., Roeyers, H., Hartman, C., Mulder, E., & Sergeant, J. (2004). Can the Children's Communication Checklist differentiate between children with autism, children with ADHD, and normal controls? *Journal of Child Psychology and Psychiatry, 45*, 1437–1453.

Dalebout, S. S., Nelson, N. W., Hletko, P. J., & Frentheway, B. (1991). Selective attention and children with ADHD; Effects of repeated measurement with and without methylphenidate. *Language, Speech, and Hearing Services in Schools, 22*, 219–227.

Edwards, W. (2002). *Mental retardation: definition, classification, and systems of supports*. Washington, DC: AAMR.

Elliot, D., Huizinga, D., & Menard, S. (1989). *Multiple problem youth: Delinquency, substance use, and mental health problems*. NY: Springer-Verlag.

Fey, M. (1991). *Language intervention with young children*. Needham Heights, MA: Allyn & Bacon.

Fletcher, J. M., Aram, D., Shaywitz, S. E., & Shaywitz, B. A. (2000). Learning, language and attention disorders in children: Comorbidity, assessment, & intervention. In P. J. Accardo & T. A. Blandis (Eds.), *Attention Deficits and Hyperactivity in Children & Adults* (pp. 241–256). NY: Marcel Dekker.

Flexer, C., Wray, D., & Ireland, J. A. (1989). Preferential seating is not enough: Issues in classroom management of hearing-impaired students. *Language, Speech, and Hearing Services in Schools, 20*, 11–21.

Flory, K., Milich, R., Lorch, E. P., Hayden, A. N., Strange, C., & Welsh, R. (2006). Online story comprehension among children with ADHD: Which core deficits are involved? *Journal of Abnormal Child Psychology, 34*, 850–862.

Gaub, M., & Carlson, C.L. (1997). Gender differences in ADHD: A meta-analysis of analysis and critical review. *Journal of the American Academy of Child and Adolescent Psychiatry, 36*, 1036–1045.

Gershon, J. (2002). A meta-analytic review of gender differences in ADHD. *Journal of Attention Disorders, 5*, 143–154.

Giddan, J. J., & Milling, L. (2000). ADHD in young children. In L. Watson, E. Crais, & T. Layton (Eds.), *Handbook of early language impairment in children*. Albany, NY: Delmar.

Gresham, F. M., & Elliot, S. N. (1990). *Social Skills Rating System*. Circle Pines, MN: American Guidance Service.

Hedberg, N. L., & Westby, C. E. (1993). *Analyzing storytelling skills: Theory to practice*. Tucson, AZ: Communication Skill Builders.

Helland, W., Biringer, E., Helland, T., & Heimann, M. (2012). Exploring language profiles for children with ADHD and children with Asperger Syndrome. *Journal of Attention Disorders, 16*, 34–43.

Helland, W., & Heimann, M. (2007). Assessment of pragmatic language impairment in children referred to psychiatric services: A pilot study of the Children's Communication Checklist in a Norwegian sample. *Logopedics Phoniatrics Vocology, 32*, 23–30.

Heyer, J. L. (1995). The responsibilities of SLPs toward children with ADHD. *Seminars in Speech & Language, 16*, 275–288.

Hughes, D., McGillivray, L., & Schmidek, M. (1997). *Guide to Narrative Language: Procedures for Assessment*. Eau Claire, WI: Thinking Publications.

Im-bolter, N., Cohen, N., & Farnia, F. (2013). I thought we were good: Social cognition, figurative language, and psychopathology. *Journal of Child Psychology and Psychiatry*. https://doi.org/10.1111/jcpp.12067

Jadad, A. R., Boyle, M., & Cunningham, C. (1999). *Treatment of attention deficit/hyperactivity disorder: Evidence report/technology assessment no. 11*. Rockville, MD: Agency for Healthcare Research & Quality, No. 00-E005.

Javorsky, J. (1996). An examination of youth with attention deficit/hyperactivity disorder and language learning disabilities: A clinical study. *Journal of Learning Disabilities, 29*(3), 247–258.

Jensen, P. (2001). Findings from the NIMH Multimodal Treatment Study of ADHD (MTA): Implications and Applications for Primary Care Providers. *Developmental and Behavioral Pediatrics, 22(1)*, 60–73.

Ketelaars, M., Cuperus, J., Jansonius, K., & Verhoeven, L. (2010). Pragmatic language impairment and associated behavioural problems. *International Journal of Language and Communication Disorders, 45*, 204–214.

Kim, O. H., & Kaiser, A. P. (2000). Language characteristics of children with ADHD. *Communication Disorders Quarterly, 21*, 154–165.

Leonard, M., Milich, R., & Lorch, P. (2011). The role of pragmatic language use in mediating the relation between hyperactivity and inattention and social skills problems. *Journal of Speech, Language, and Hearing Research, 54*, 567–579.

Lienemann, T. O., & Reid, R. (2008). Using self-regulated strategy development to improve expository writing with students with Attention Deficit Hyperactivity Disorder. *Exceptional Children, 74*(4), 471–486.

Lindsay, G., & Dockrell, J.E. (2008). Outcomes for young people with a history of specific language impairment at 16–17 years: A more positive picture? In V. Joffe, M. Cruice, & S. Chiat (Eds.), *Language disorder in children and adults: New issues in research and practice* (pp. 138–159). Hoboken, NJ: John Wiley & Sons.

Lindsay, G., Dockrell, J., & Strand, S. (2007). Longitudinal patterns of behaviour problems in children with specific speech and language difficulties: Child and contextual factors. *British Journal of Educational Psychology, 77*(4), 811–828.

Lorch, E. P., Diener, M. B., Can den Broek, P., Sanchez, R. P., Milich, R., & Welsh, R. (1999). The effects of story structure on the recall of stories in children with attention deficit hyperactivity disorder. *Journal of Education Psychology, 91*(2), 273–283.

Love, A. J., & Thompson, M. G. (1988). Language disorders and attention deficit disorders in young children referred for psychiatric services: Analysis of prevalence and a conceptual synthesis. *American Journal of Orthopsychiatry, 58*(1), 52–64.

Mace, F. C., Belfiore, R. J., & Hutchinson, M. (2001). Operant theory and research on self-regulation. In B. Zimmerman & D. Schunk (Eds.), *Learning and academic achievement: Theoretical perspectives* (pp. 39–65). Mahwah, NJ: Lawrence Erlbaum.

Mann, E. M., Ikeda, Y., Mueller, C. W., Takahashi, A., Tao, K. T., Humris, E., et al. (1992). Cross-cultural differences in rating hyperactive-disruptive behaviors in children. *American Journal of Psychiatry, 149*, 1539–1542.

McGoey, K. E., Eckert, T. L., & DuPaul, G. (2002). Early intervention for preschool-age children with ADHD: A literature review. *Journal of Emotional Behavioral Disorders, 10*, 14–28.

McInnes, A., Humphries, T., Hogg-Johnson, S., & Tannock, R. (2003). Listening comprehension and working memory are impaired in attention-deficit hyperactivity disorder. *Journal of Abnormal Child Psychology, 31*(4), 427–443.

McNamara, J. K., Willoughby, T., Chalmers, H., & YLC-CURA. (2005). Psychosocial status of adolescents with learning disabilities with and without comorbid attention deficit hyperactivity disorder. *Learning Disabilities Research and Practice, 20*(4), 234–244.

MTA Cooperative Group. (1999a). A 14-month randomized clinical trial of treatment strategies for attention-deficit hyperactivity disorder. *Archives of General Psychiatry, 56*, 1073–1086.

MTA Cooperative Group. (1999b). Effects of co-morbid anxiety, poverty, session attendance, and community medication on treatment outcome in children with attention-deficit hyperactivity disorder. *Archives of General Psychiatry, 56*, 1088–1096.

Mueller, C. W., Mann, E. M., Thanapum, S., Humris, E., Ikeda, Y., Takahashi, A., et al. (1995). Teachers' ratings of disruptive behavior in five countries. *Journal of Clinical Child Psychology, 24*, 434–442.

National Institute of Mental Health (2000). *NIMH research on treatment for attention deficit hyperactivity disorder (ADHD): The multimodal treatment study— questions and answers*. [online]. Available: http://www.nimh.nih.gov/childhp/mtaqa.cfm

Nilsen, E. S., Mangal, L., & MacDonald, K. (2013). Referential communication in children with ADHD: Challenges in the role of a listener. *Journal of Speech, Language, and Hearing Research, 56*, 590–603.

Pastor, P. S., & Reuben, C. A. (2008). Diagnosed ADHD and learning disability: US 2004–2006. National Center for Health Statistics. *Vital Health Stat, 10*(237). http://www.cdc.gov/mnchs/data/series/sr_10/SR10-237.pdf

Pelc, K., Kornreich, C., Foisy, M.-L., & Bernard, D. (2006). Recognition of emotional facial expressions in attention deficit hyperactivity disorder. *Pediatric Neurology, 35*, 93–97.

Pelham, W. E., & Hoza, B. (1996). Intensive treatment: A summer treatment program for children with ADHD. In E. Hibbs & H. Jensen (Eds.), *Psychosocial treatment for child and adolescent disorders: Empirically based strategies for clinical practice* (pp. 311–340). New York: American Psychological Association Press.

Pelham, W. E., Wheeler, T., & Chronis, A. (1998). Empirically supported psychosocial treatments for attention deficit hyperactivity disorders. *Journal of Clinical Child Psychology, 27*, 190–205.

Pisecco, S., Baker, D. B., Silva, P. A., & Brooke, M. (2001). Boys with reading disabilities and/or ADHD: Distinctions in Early Childhood. *Journal of Learning Disabilities, 34*(2), 98–106.

Rapport, M. D., Stoner, G., & Jones, J. T. (1986). Comparing classroom and clinic measures of attention deficit disorder: Differential, idiosyncratic, and dose- response effects of methylphenidate. *Journal of Counseling and Clinical Psychology, 54*, 334–341.

Re, A. M., Pedron, M., & Cornoldi, C. (2007). Expressive writing difficulties in children described as exhibiting ADHD symptoms. *Journal of Learning Disabilities, 40*(3), 244–255.

Redmond, S. M., & Rice, M. L. (2002). Stability of behavioral ratings of children with specific language impairment. *Journal of Speech, Language, and Hearing Research, 45*, 190–201.

Reid, R., DuPaul, G. J., Power, T. J., Anastopoulos, A. D., Rogers-Adkinson, D., Noll, M. B., & Riccio, C. (1998). Assessing culturally different students for attention deficit hyperactivity disorder using behavior rating scales. *Journal of Abnormal Child Psychology, 26*, 187–198.

Reid, R., Trout, A. L., & Schartz, M. (2005). Self-regulation interventions for children with ADHD. *Exceptional Children, 71*(4), 361–378.

Renz, K., Lorch, E. P., Milich, R., Lemberger, C., Bodner, A., & Welsh, R. (2003). Online story representation in boys with attention deficit hyperactivity disorder. *Journal of Abnormal Child Psychology, 31*, 93–104.

Rescorla, L., Ross, G. S., & McClure, S. (2007). Language delay and behavioral/ emotional problems in toddlers: Findings from two developmental clinics. *Journal of Speech, Language, and Hearing Research, 50*, 1063–1078.

Retherford, K. S. (2000). *Guide to Analysis of Language Transcripts* (3rd ed.). Eau Claire, WI: Thinking Publications.

St. Clair, C., Pickles, A., Durkin, K., & Conti-Ramsden, G. (2011). A longitudinal study of behavioral, emotional and social difficulties in individuals with a history of specific language impairment (SLI). *Journal of Communication Disorders, 44*(2), 186–199.

Sonuga-Barke, E., Minocha, K., Taylor, E., & Sandberg, S. (1993). Inter-ethnic bias in teachers' ratings of childhood hyperactivity. *British Journal of Developmental Psychology, 11*, 187–200.

Starck, M., Grunwald, J., & Schlarb, A. A. (2016). Occurrence of ADHD in parents of ADHD children in a clinical sample. *Neuropsychiatric Disease and Treatment, 12*, 581–588.

Storebo, O.J., Ramstad, E., Krogh, H.B., Nilausen T.D., Skoog, M., Homskov, M., … Gould, C. (2015). Methylphenidate for children and adolescents with ADHD. *Cochrane Database of Systematic Reviews 2015*, Issue aa, Art. No.: CD009885. https://doi.org/10.1002/14651858.CD009885.pub

Tetnowski, J. A. (2004). ADHD and concomitant communicative disorders. *Seminars in Speech & Language, 25*(3), 215–224.

Tetter, P. A. (1998). *Interventions for ADHD: Treatment in developmental contexts*. New York: Guilford Press.

Trautman, R. C., Giddan, J. J., & Jurs, S. G. (1990). Language risk factor in emotionally disturbed children within a school and day treatment program. *Journal of Childhood Communication Disorders, 13*(2), 123–133.

U.S. Department of Education (US DOE). (2003). *Identifying and treating attention deficit hyperactivity disorder: A resource for school and home*. Washington, DC: DOE.

Valera, E. M., & Seidman, L. J. (2006). Neurobiology of ADHD in preschoolers. *Infants and Young Children, 19*(2), 94–108.

Visser, S.N., Danielson, M.L., Bitsko, R.H., Holbrook, JR., Kogan, M.D., Ghandour, R.M. et al. (2014). Trends in the parent report of health care provider-diagnosed and medicated ADHD: US, 2003–2011. J. *American Academy of Child and Adolescent Psychiatry, 53*(1), 34–46.e2.

Visser, S. N., Zablotsky, B., Holbrook, J. R., Danielson, M. L., & Bitsko, R. H. (2015). Diagnostic experience of children with Attention-deficit/Hyperactivity Disorder. *National Health Statistics Reports, 81*, 1–8.

Walkup, J. T., Stossel, L., & Rendleman, R. (2014). Beyond rising rates: Personalised medicine and public health approaches to the diagnosis and treatment of ADHD. *Journal of American Academy of Child & Adolescent Psychiatry, 53*(1), 14–16.

Weaver, C. (1993). Understanding and educating students with attention deficit/hyperactivity disorder: Toward a system theory and whole language perspective. *American Journal of Speech-Language Pathology, 2*, 79–89.

Westby, C. E., & Cutler, S. K. (1994). Language and ADHD: Understanding the bases and treatment of self-regulatory deficits. *Topics in Language Disorders, 14*, 58–76.

Whitehouse, A. J. O., Robinson, M., & Zubrick, S. R. (2011). Late talking and the risk for psychosocial problems during childhood and adolescence. *Pediatrics, 128*(2), 324–332.

Willcutt, E. G. (2012). The prevalence of DSM-IV attention-deficit/hyperactivity disorder: A meta-analytic review. *Neurotherapeutics, 9*, 490–499.

Willinger, U., Brunner, E., Diendorfer-Radner, G., Mag, J. S., Sirsch, U., & Eisenwort, B. (2003). Behavior in children with language development disorders. *Canadian Journal of Psychiatry, 48*, 607–614.

Chapter 12
Children with Autism Spectrum Disorders

Introduction

Autism spectrum disorder (ASD) is a common childhood disorder with core deficits in social communication and behavior. Currently, it is a behavioral disorder defined by its clinical manifestations, but research indicates it is a brain disorder with a genetic basis and an increased occurrence in twins and subsequent siblings (Bailey, Luthert, Dean, Harding, & Janota, 1998; Barton & Volkmar, 1998; Edelson, 2015; Geschwind, 2011). Although advances in genetic testing are identifying specific gene locations linked to autism, the search continues as more than 100 rare or uncommon single genes are associated with autism (Coe, Girirajan, & Eichler, 2012; Neale et al., 2012; O'Roak et al., 2012; Sanders et al., 2012).

Incidence rates remain high at 1 in 68 (Christensen et al., 2016) but are unchanged from the 2014 Centers for Disease Control (CDC) reports based on available health and education records for 8-year-old children. This rate is higher, however, than the 2012 CDC reports of 1 in 88. Diagnosis in males continues to predominate with some suspicion that girls are identified later than boys (Giarelli et al., 2010). Because recent reports indicate significant increases in ASD diagnoses in some communities with percentages of children diagnosed varying wildly, it remains unclear whether the overall percentage of children diagnosed with ASD has stabilized or continues to increase. In those communities where both health and education records were available for review as opposed to just health records, incidence rates were the highest. This suggests that schools play a critical role in assessing and supporting children with ASD. Interestingly, records documented developmental concerns by age 3, yet less than 50% of the children eventually diagnosed with ASD received a comprehensive assessment by 3. This delay in diagnosis also meant a delay in services.

Some important findings related to diagnosis were identified for different cultural groups even though the research suggests there is no difference in risk of

P. A. Prelock, T. L. Hutchins, *Clinical Guide to Assessment and Treatment of Communication Disorders*, Best Practices in Child and Adolescent Behavioral Health Care, https://doi.org/10.1007/978-3-319-93203-3_12

ASD across cultures. Christensen et al. (2015) found that black and Hispanic children are identified with ASD less often than non-Hispanic white children and when they are identified, their comprehensive evaluations occur later than those for white children.

The speech-language pathologist (SLP) is an important partner with families, physicians, psychologists, and other related health and educational professionals in the diagnosis, assessment, and treatment of children with ASD. Because a primary core deficit is in the area of social communication and social interaction, the SLP has a significant role to play. This chapter will summarize the core deficit areas for making a diagnosis, highlight some of the relevant comorbidities, identify early indicators or markers of autism, explain the specific communication challenges that characterize children with ASD, and describe the basic assessment and intervention needs for children with ASD emphasizing the role of communication and the SLP.

Diagnosis and Comorbidities

The DSM-5 (American Psychiatric Association, APA, 2013) describes two core deficit areas in the diagnosis of children with ASD. First, children must currently demonstrate or by history show persistent challenges in social communication and social interaction. Second, children must currently demonstrate or by history exhibit restricted, repetitive patterns of behavior, interests, or activities. There are three components of the social communication and social interaction core deficit area including (1) impairments in social emotional reciprocity (i.e., abnormal social approach, failure in back and forth conversation, reduced sharing of interests, emotions or affect, failure to initiate or respond to social interaction), (2) impairments in nonverbal communication behaviors during social interactions (i.e., poorly integrated verbal and nonverbal communication, abnormal eye contact and body language, deficits in understanding and using gestures, lack of facial expressions and nonverbal communication), and (3) impairments in understanding, developing, and maintaining relationships (i.e., difficulties adjusting behavior to different social contexts, problems in sharing imaginative play, challenges making friends, and lack of interest in peers) (APA, 2013). There are four components of the restricted, repetitive patterns core deficit area including (1) stereotyped or repetitive motor movements, use of objects, or speech (i.e., simple motor stereotypies, lining up toys or flipping objects, echolalia, idiosyncratic phrases); (2) insistence on sameness, inflexible adherence to routines, or ritualized patterns of verbal and nonverbal behaviors (i.e., extreme distress with small changes, difficulty with transitions, rigid thinking patterns and greeting rituals, needing to take same route or eat the same food every day); (3) highly restricted, fixated interests abnormal in intensity or focus (i.e., strong attachment to or preoccupation with unusual objects, excessively circumscribed or perseverative interests); and (4) hyper- or hypo activity to sensory input or unusual interest in sensory aspects of the environment (i.e., indifference to pain/temperature, adverse response to specific sounds or textures, excessive smelling or touching of objects, visual fascination with lights or movement) (APA, 2013).

When making a diagnosis of autism, several conditions must be met. First, the child must demonstrate all three components of the social communication and social interaction deficit. Second, the child must exhibit at least two of the components of the restricted, repetitive patterns of behavior, interests, or activities. Third, the observed symptoms must be present in the early developmental period and cause significant impairments in social, occupational, or other areas of function. Fourth, the observed deficits cannot be more appropriately explained by an intellectual disability (ID) or global developmental delay. Fifth, further assessment must be done to determine if the child has ASD with or without an accompanying intellectual and/or language impairment. Finally, if an associated medical, genetic, or environmental factor or if another neurodevelopment, psychiatric, or behavioral disorder is identified, this information must be specified. Notably, ASD and ID can co-occur, but social communication would be below the expected developmental level. Further, children with social communication deficits who do not meet the criteria for ASD would be assessed for a social communication disorder.

The DSM-5 identifies the level of severity for children diagnosed with ASD based on the type of support they will require and aligns severity and support level to the core deficit areas. Table 12.1 provides a summary of the severity levels with examples of what that might look like in a child with social communication deficits and restricted repetitive behaviors.

There are some concerns with the application of the new criteria for ASD in the DSM-5 as compared to the DSM-IV. Results are mixed for the percentage of children with Pervasive Developmental Disorders-Not Otherwise Specified (PDD-NOS) and Asperger Syndrome who meet the ASD criteria in the DSM-5, but generally those with higher skills were less likely to meet all three social communication and social interaction criteria (Smith, Reichow, & Volkmar, 2015; Young & Rodi, 2014). It is still too early to determine the real impact of the change in criteria on diagnosis, but the intent is to ensure that children who may not qualify using the DSM-5 criteria will still receive the needed supports.

When considering co-occurring diagnoses, the CDC indicated that about 4 in 1,000 children 8 years of age who had ASD also had an intellectual disability (ID) with a greater male to female prevalence (Christensen et al., 2016). In children who are deaf and hard of hearing with ASD, the prevalence rate of ID is 15.5% compared to 8.2% who are deaf without ASD (Szymanski, Brice, Lam, & Hotto, 2012). Notably, comorbid ASD and ID are significantly lower in non-Hispanic white children than in non-Hispanic black children (Christensen et al., 2016).

SLPs often receive referrals for children with communication delays or deficits in social functioning which may signal an ASD, ID, or other condition. When making a differential diagnosis, the SLP is usually part of a team with experience in recognizing the similarities and differences between ASD and ID. Table 12.2 presents a summary of the similarities and differences among the two conditions.

Table 12.1 Severity levels for deficits in social communication/social interaction and restricted repetitive patterns of behavior, interests, or activities

Severity level	Social communication (SC)/Social interaction (SI)	Restricted, repetitive patterns of behavior, interests, or activities
Level 3: Requiring very substantial support	Severe deficits in verbal (V) and nonverbal (NV) SC cause: Severe impairments in functioning Very limited initiation of social interactions Minimal response to social overtures from others *Example*: child with few words of intelligible speech who rarely initiates interaction, makes unusual approaches to meet needs only, and responds to only very direct social approaches	Inflexibility Extreme difficulty coping with change Restricted/repetitive behaviors markedly interfere with functioning in all spheres Great distress/difficulty changing focus or action
Level 2: Requiring substantial support	Marked deficits in V and NV SC Social impairments apparent even with supports in place Limited initiation of SI Reduced or abnormal responses to social overtures from others *Example:* child speaks in simple sentences, with interaction limited to narrow special interests, using markedly odd NV communication	Inflexibility Difficulty coping with change Restricted/repetitive behaviors appear frequently enough to be obvious to the casual observer and interfere with functioning in a variety of contexts Distress/difficulty changing focus or action
Level 1: Requiring support	With supports in place, deficits in SC cause noticeable impairments: Difficulty initiating social interactions Atypical or unsuccessful responses to social overtures of others Decreased interest in SI *Example*: child speaks in full sentences and engages in communication, but reciprocal conversation with others fails, and attempts to make friends are odd and typically unsuccessful	Inflexibility causes significant interference with functioning in one or more contexts Problems of organization and planning hamper independence

Adapted from APA (2013)

Table 12.2 Similarities and differences between ASD and ID

Similarities	Differences
Onset during the developmental period	Children with ASD have a range of intellectual abilities, while children with ID always have deficits in intellectual functioning
Deficits in nonverbal and verbal communication skills	Children with ASD don't follow a typical developmental progression, while children with ID develop skills at a slower rate but usually follow patterns of typical development
Challenges in social interaction	Children with ASD have theory of mind (ToM) difficulties regardless of their intellectual functioning, and ToM impairments are more severe and likely different in nature in children with ASD compared to children with ID alone
Attention and academic challenges	Children with ASD will have a range of abilities, and not all children with ASD will have the level of deficits a child with ID might have in these areas

Table 12.3 Characteristics of ASD and other developmental disabilities

Autism spectrum disorders (ASD)	Other developmental disorders
Language	*Developmental language disorders*
Impaired pragmatics and prosody	Spared pragmatics
Unusual word choices	Limited vocabulary
Minor impairments in grammar and speech production	Impaired grammar and speech production and poor intelligibility
Abnormal use of scripts, questions, and perseverative comments	Few abnormal features
Poorer comprehension than expression	Better comprehension than expression
Poorer gesture use and integration of gestures and verbalizations	More likely to respond in natural contexts
Lack spontaneous pretend play	Uses some conventional gestures
Poorer adaptive skills	Spontaneously demonstrates pretend play
Attention	*ADHD/ADD*
Poor joint attention	Variable inattention
Highly attentive in self-selected activities	Restless, fidgety, and impulsive
Sensorimotor issues	*Tics/Tourette's syndrome, OCD*
Frequent stereotypies	Rapid and irregular tics
Increased or decreased response to sensory stimuli	Compulsive touching
Some self-injurious behavior	Little self-injurious behavior
Decreases with age	Varies over time

Adapted from Paul and Fahim (2014), Rapin and Tuchman (2008), Ventola et al. (2007)

In addition to ID, there are other developmental disabilities that may share characteristics of ASD. Table 12.3 provides a summary of the language, attention, and sensory characteristics of ASD as compared to other neurodevelopmental disorders that may co-occur or require a differential diagnosis (Rapin & Tuchman, 2008). The SLP can be particularly helpful in parsing out the language and attention challenges of children with ASD and other disorders.

Identification and Assessment of Early Indicators for ASD

Two approaches have been used in the literature to examine potential early markers for autism. The first approach is retrospective video review of children who are already diagnosed with ASD, but videos taken of their early development are revisited to determine if there are behaviors in the first 2 years of life that differentiate them from typical peers or peers with other neurodevelopmental disabilities. Research using this approach has consistently identified a failure to point, orient to name, show objects, and respond to or initiate joint attention (Baranek, 1999; Clifford, Young & Williamson, 2007; Mars, Mauk, & Dowrick, 1998; Osterling & Dawson, 1994; Werner, Dawson, Osterling & Dinno, 2000). A review of all videotaped studies assessing early markers of ASD indicated the most common indicators across studies included less response to name, less looking at others, poorer eye contact in both quality and frequency, and less positive facial expressions and intersubjective behaviors like showing shared attention (St. Georges et al., 2010).

The second approach is prospective and includes early screenings and follow-up for at-risk populations to determine if a diagnosis is made and what might be predictive at 12, 18, 24, and 36 months of age (Baird et al., 2000; Baron-Cohen, Allen & Gillberg, 1992; Baron-Cohen et al., 1996; Dietz, Swinkels, van Daalen, van Engeland, & Buitelaar, 2006; Kleinman et al., 2008; Lord, 1995; Robins, Fein, Barton, & Green 2001; Shumway, Wetherby & Woods, 2003; Wetherby & Woods, 2002, 2003; Wetherby et al., 2004). These studies have resulted in the development of several screening tools frequently used by SLPs who are often the first professional to see a child with or at risk for ASD. These screening measures can also be used by primary healthcare providers to determine when it might be appropriate to make a referral for a more comprehensive evaluation. Table 12.4 provides a description of the most frequently used tools to screen early markers of ASD.

In her prospective assessment of young children at risk for ASD, Lord (1995) found that the clearest discriminators for 2-year-old children included directing attention (showing, pointing, vocalizing, etc.) and attention to voice (particularly neutral voice), while the clearest discriminators for 3-year-old children involved seeking to share enjoyment (best predictor), pointing to express interest (more refined form of directing attention), using another's body as a tool (hand leading), unusual hand and finger mannerisms, and attention to voice. In a more recent prospective study, Ozonoff et al. (2010) found that frequency of eye gaze (to faces), social smiles, and directed vocalizations were comparable to typically developing children at 6 months, but differences in the frequency of these behaviors occurred by 12 months – discriminating those children who eventually received a diagnosis of ASD.

To probe a child's early social skills and language at 12 months, the following strategies would be appropriate and may help determine the need for further referral if a primary healthcare provider does not have access to the screening tools outlined in Table 12.4 (Johnson, 2008; Johnson, Myers, & Council on Children with Disabilities, 2007):

- Assess child's ability to follow a point by saying: "Look! See the ____" while pointing to an interesting object in sight or a picture on wall; if no response, say the child's name or tap the child's shoulder and repeat the "Look . . .".
- Call out the child's name and assess whether the child turns and connects; there should be a response by the second attempt.
- Ask the parents about the child's favorite toys, how the child plays, and how much the child engages in solitary play.
- Ask the parents if their child looks at them when speaking, babbles, waves bye, attends to their voice or other environmental sounds, makes unusual vocalizations, or laughs inappropriately.

If a child lacks an appropriate gaze, does not use joyful expressions with their gaze, has poor or absent reciprocal vocalization patterns, attends to environmental sounds but not vocalizations, fails to recognize familiar voices, is not babbling or is delayed in babbling, fails to use gestures (e.g., waving, pointing, showing), and

Table 12.4 Summary of ASD screening tools for infants and toddlers

Screening tool	Relevant literature	Items predictive of ASD
Checklist for Autism in Toddlers (CHAT) http://www.chat.com	Baron-Cohen, Allen, and Gillberg (1992, 1996)	Failure to point to express interest (protodeclarative pointing) Failure to show interest in or joint attention for pleasure or connection with another (gaze monitoring) Failure to demonstrate symbolic play (pretend play)
Modified Checklist for Autism in Toddlers (M-CHAT) http://www.mchatscreen.com	Robins et al. (2001), Kleinman et al. (2008), Scarpa et al. (2013)	Lack of pointing Failure to respond to name Lack of interest in other children Failure to "show" objects Inability to follow a point Failure to imitate another
Systematic Observation of Red Flags for ASD (SORF)	Shumway et al. (2003) Wetherby and Woods (2002, 2003), Wetherby et al. (2004)	Lack of appropriate eye gaze Warm, joyful expressions with gaze Sharing enjoyment or interest Response to name Showing Coordination of gaze, facial expression, gesture, and sound Demonstration of unusual prosody Repetitive movements or posturing of body, arms, hands, or fingers Repetitive movements with objects Key indicators: social communication and repetitive behaviors
Early Screening of Autistic Traits Questionnaire (ESAT)	Dietz et al. (2006)	Interest in people Smiles directly Reacts when spoken to
Quantitative Checklist for Autism in Toddler (Q-CHAT)	Allison et al. (2008), Allison, Auyeung, and Baron-Cohen (2012)	Not reported as it is a dimensional screening tool
Communication Symbolic Behavior Scales-Developmental Profile (CSBS-DP)	Shumway and Wetherby (2009)	Lower rate of communicative acts Lower proportion of joint attention Fewer deictic gestures and more primitive gestures
Parents Observation of Early Markers Scale (POEMS)	Feldman et al. (2012)	Greater social and communication challenges Difficulty with waiting
Baby and Infant Screen for Children with Autism Traits (BISCUIT: Part 1)	Matson, Wilkins, and Fodstad (2011), Kozlowski, Matson, Worley, Sipes, and Horovitz (2012)	Greater social and communication challenges

lacks interest or response to neutral statements, then it is likely you are seeing early indicators of ASD, and an immediate referral should be made for a comprehensive assessment (Johnson et al., 2007).

Language, Communication, and Social Interaction Challenges in ASD

Young children with ASD use fewer gestures (e.g., nodding or shaking their head), display more echolalia and stereotyped phrases, and are less likely to initiate and respond to verbal communication than other children with developmental disabilities (Lord, 1995; Mildenberger, Sitter, Noterdaeme, & Amorosa, 2001; Trillingsgaard, Sorensen, Nemec, & Jorgensen, 2005). Children with ASD are also less likely to coordinate their vocalizations, make eye gaze with their communicative partners, or use gestures. Their poorer rate of communicative acts is a strong predictor of language outcome at 3 years (Shumway & Wetherby, 2009).

Receptive language is often more impaired than expressive language, and the tendency of children with ASD to be more attentive to sights and sounds in their environment impacts their expressive language development and language comprehension (Bopp, Mirenda, & Zumbo, 2009). Articulation is often normal in children with ASD, and syntax usually develops following the same chronology as typically developing children matched for mental age. Children with ASD often use the same word categories as those who are typically developing; but some word categories are used less often (e.g., cognitive states like think, know, remember, pretend), and many use words with special meanings. Confusion with personal pronouns (e.g., mixing the terms "you" and "me") and intonational peculiarities is also common (Kim, Paul, Tager-Flusberg, & Lord, 2014).

Joint Attention Toddlers with ASD are more impaired in joint attention, imitation, empathic responses, pointing to express interest, interest in other children, and displaying a range of facial expressions compared to children with other developmental disabilities (DD) (Dawson et al., 2004; Lord, 1995; Rogers, Hepburn, Stackhouse, & Wehner, 2003; Trillingsgaard et al., 2005). Joint attention, which requires a child to show interest in or connection with another, is a pivotal skill for later language learning but is a frequent area of deficit for young children with ASD (Bakeman & Adamson, 1984; Baron-Cohen, 1987; Loveland & Landry, 1986). Joint attention deficits are found by the second year of life in children with ASD and are typically characterized by poor affect and eye contact (Clifford & Dissanayake, 2008). Related to their deficits in joint attention, young children with ASD appear more interested in familiar objects than people when compared to typically developing children and children with Down syndrome (Adamson, Deckner, & Bakeman, 2010). Notably, joint attention is a strong predictor of concurrent language ability (Wetherby, Watt, Morgan, & Shumway, 2007). A child's lack of joint attention impacts their ability to acquire new words and develop their vocabulary as they are missing opportunities to enter a joint attentional focus with an adult (Kasari, Freeman, & Paparella, 2001; Tomasello, 1995). Children with ASD who are able to respond to joint attention bids have higher language scores and greater language gains over time including an increased mean length of utterance and better receptive language (Bono, Daley & Sigman, 2004; Murray et al., 2008). As children with ASD increase in age, deficits in joint attention may impact their ability to participate in cooperative language and academic tasks (Colombi et al., 2009).

Social Interaction When considering the reciprocal social interactions of children with ASD, their social communication difficulties become evident. Children with ASD are less likely to greet using spontaneous verbal and nonverbal gestures and may not establish eye contact during their greetings (Hobson & Lee, 1998). Although they may respond to caregivers who are making active attempts to engage them, they vary in the manner and frequency with which they initiate attempts at interaction (Hauck, Fein, Waterhouse, & Feinstein, 1995). Their communicative attempts are often unconventional and involve a limited range of communicative partners with a tendency to pursue interactions with caregivers more than strangers (Mundy & Sigman, 1989; Sigman & Ungerer, 1984; Sigman, Ungerer, Mundy, & Sherman, 1987), adults more than peers (Lord & Magill, 1989), in structured more than unstructured contexts, and in environments with less complexity (Baron-Cohen, 1987; Lewis & Boucher, 1988; Jarrold, Boucher, & Smith, 1993).

Theory of Mind Children and adolescents with ASD demonstrate a number of theory of mind challenges that impact both their social communication and social interaction, including but not limited to the following:

- Establishing joint attention and playing symbolically
- Recognizing and understanding emotions
- Adjusting one's behavior to accommodate a particular situation
- Planning one's own behavior and recognizing the plans of others
- Predicting behavior
- Inferring mental states
- Understanding deception
- Recognizing false beliefs

The impact of these deficits is far-reaching and is a unique challenge area for children with ASD. For example, children with ASD are less likely than other children including children with Down syndrome to talk about the mental states of characters in pictures or stories (Baron-Cohen, Leslie, & Frith, 1986). Preadolescents with high cognitive and linguistic skills do not differ from typical peers on overall production of mental state terms (e.g., desire, emotion, cognition) but do differ in their production of personal narratives (Bang, Burns, & Nadig, 2013). Children with ASD generally recognize emotions of happy, sad, and mad but are less likely to recognize fear and other more complex emotions (Uljarevic & Hamilton, 2013). Children with ASD and a mental age well above 4 years of age fail false-belief tasks that are passed by children with Down syndrome and children without disabilities at age 4 as they seem to have a poor cognitive capacity to represent the internal beliefs, feelings, and thoughts of others (Mundy, Sigman & Kasari, 1990).

Knowing that theory of mind is also a core area of deficit for children with ASD, it is important to understand the social emotions of children with ASD. This requires a self-conscious ability to put oneself in the place of another and creates greater complexity in social understanding for children with ASD (Kasari, Chamberlain & Bauminger, 2001). For example, 8- to 14-year-old children with ASD report feelings of pride and understand conditions that elicit pride as often as typically developing children (Kasari, Sigman, Baumgartner, & Stipek, 1993); however, they include references to pride less often in pictorial representations of situations designed to elicit pride and describe "happy" vs. "proud." They also take longer to recall examples of pride and are generally nonspecific in their examples which is similar to their understanding and descriptions of embarrassment and guilt (Capps, Yirmiya, & Sigman, 1992). Empathy is another emotion that challenges children with ASD as they perform less well on labeling emotions of protagonists and on identifying empathy compared to typically developing children (Yirmiya et al., 1992).

Higher cognitive abilities appear to be associated with better performance on social-emotion measures in children with ASD but not for those who are typically developing (Kasari et al., 2001). Importantly, though, fewer social experiences and reciprocal interactions with others affect the development of social emotions in ASD. Children with ASD may take longer to describe an experience with social emotions or give less personal-related examples and often compensate by providing memorized answers that do not reflect an actual feeling or experience. Providers can access the Theory of Mind Atlas (ToMA) as a resource to read more about different aspects of theory of mind (see www.theoryofmindinventory.com).

Assessment Considerations

Assessment for children with ASD requires a team approach, including the parents and other primary caregivers, educational professionals who work with the child, and a healthcare team experienced in the diagnosis of ASD. Because of the unique deficit areas in social communication and social interaction as well as behavior, and the associated health conditions in ASD, a physician (e.g., developmental pediatrician, child psychiatrist or child neurologist), a psychologist, and a speech-language pathologist are critical members of an assessment team.

The gold standards for assessment are the *Autism Diagnostic Observation Schedule-2* (ADOS-2) as a child measure and the *Autism Diagnostic Interview-Revised* as a parent-informant measure (ADI-R). The ADOS-2 (Lord, Rutter, et al., 2013) is made up of four modules used to assess children through adults and a toddler module for 12- to 30-month-olds (Lord, Luyster, Gotham & Guthrie, 2013). The ADOS-2 is an observational, semi-structured standardized tool used to assess the communication, interaction, play, and restricted and repetitive behaviors of children with or suspected of having ASD. The ADI-R (Lord, Rutter & Le Couteur, 1994) is used with the primary caregiver and focuses on three areas: (1) reciprocal social interaction, greeting, emotional sharing, offering and seeking comfort, and developing friendships; (2) communication and language, social language use, conversational discourse, idiosyncratic language, and stereotyped utterances; and (3) repetitive, restricted, and stereotyped behaviors, preoccupations, abnormal attachments, rituals, and unusual sensory needs. Although originally developed for children from 5 years through early adulthood (with a mental age of at least 2 years), new algorithms have been applied to existing research databases with toddlers and young preschoolers, from 12 to 47 months down to a nonverbal age of 10 months (Kim, Thurm, Shumway, & Lord, 2013). The ADI-R should not be used in isolation but rather in conjunction with other instruments in diagnosing ASD. There are a number of other checklists and scales that are available and used to assess children suspected of exhibiting ASD, but the ADOS-2 and ADI-R are the most commonly accepted along with the clinical judgement of experienced practitioners.

Through their assessment practices, SLPs have an important role in creating profiles of social communication and social interaction strengths and challenges for children with ASD. This is crucial if a child's educational team is to implement a developmentally and individually appropriate curriculum as individualized profiles must be considered in program planning (Fernell et al., 2010). Identifying communication profiles provides the team with critical information for prioritizing communication and social interaction intervention goals. Social communication profiles can also help predict both developmental level and autism symptoms. Wetherby et al. (2007) found that comprehension was a strong predictor of developmental level, and the ability to regulate behavior and use gestures was a strong predictor of autism at 3 years of age. By 20 months, children with ASD appear to have distinct profiles of social communication (Wetherby et al., 2007) reinforcing the importance of SLPs assessing the communication strengths and challenges of young children with or at risk for ASD. It is vital, too, to create a developmental framework for a child that considers natural language samples, parental report, and standardized measures (Tager-Flusberg et al., 2009)

Interviewing those who know the child best across environments is the best place to start to obtain information that will guide program planning for a child with ASD. Most SLPs will observe a child's communication and social interaction during spontaneous exchanges in a variety of environments such as with familiar and unfamiliar adults and peers, in structured and unstructured situations, in small and large groups, and at home, school, work or in the community. A child's behavior is sampled by designing opportunities for initiating interaction; responding to attempts at interaction; requesting information from a communicative partner; commenting on an activity, event, or during an interaction; following routines; providing or offering information; and understanding requests or expectations for performance. It is important, too, to identify the contextual supports that foster or hinder a child's success such as describing the environmental arrangement, identifying the props used, and determining the level of prompts needed. Additionally, it is critical to observe the means a child uses to communicate, including identifying contact gestures (e.g., gives, shows or pushes), distal gestures (e.g., points, reaches, waves), and vocalizations (e.g., noises, cries, laughter, vowels, consonants, syllable shapes, phonetically consistent forms, etc.). Profiles for social interaction also include examining a child's ability to engage and take turns in emotionally appropriate ways (Constantino, Przybeck, Friesen & Todd, 2000); assessing the child's awareness of the emotional and interpersonal cues of others; documenting the child's attempts to avoid interaction or social encounters in familiar vs. unfamiliar contexts; and looking for the child's response to social opportunities in complex environments and reactions to different levels of stimulation. The SLP helps define the interaction features that enhance social communicative competence and through a communication profile, can identify the strengths and challenge areas for a child with ASD.

Intervention Considerations

Our challenge in intervention is understanding the worries, concerns, and needs of the family, managing our own biases about what interventions might be best for a particular child, and collaborating with the family and the child's team to select, implement, and evaluate evidence-based interventions that will support the priority goals for the child with ASD and his or her family. There are a number of approaches to intervention for children with ASD ranging from those founded in a traditional behavioral approach to those characterized by a developmental social-pragmatic approach. Behavioral approaches to intervention have significant support in the literature, and they focus on implementing the principles that explain how learning takes place. Positive reinforcement is one such principle. For example, when a response is followed by a reward, the behavior is more likely to be repeated. Through decades of research, the field of behavior analysis has developed many techniques (e.g., modeling, shaping, reinforcing) for increasing desired behaviors and reducing those that may cause harm or interfere with learning. Applied behavior analysis (ABA) is the use of these techniques and principles to bring about meaningful and positive change in behavior and establishes the basis for many ASD intervention programs. The literature, however, also recognizes that more naturalistic developmental approaches have a role in ensuring positive outcomes for children in social communication and social interaction.

There is general consensus that young children receiving a diagnosis of ASD will require intensive instruction (on average 25 hours a week) in which a child is engaged (National Research Council, NRC, 2001). Engagement activities can occur in the home, with an individual therapist, in a child care center, or in a preschool, to name some of the possible contexts. Engagement is the keyword here as it means a child is actively responding to communication attempts and initiating bids for communication. Instruction should be goal based and systematically planned with teaching opportunities occurring throughout the day using developmentally appropriate activities. Families, peers, and siblings are appropriate partners to support the child's learning maintenance and generalization, and adult support ensures sufficient scaffolding. And of course, beginning as early as possible is critical (NRC, 2001).

Although a majority of the research examines the impact of comprehensive intervention programs on outcomes for preschool children with ASD, there are some active ingredients in the intervention programs reviewed in the NRC (2001) report that can be integrated into programs for school-age children with ASD. Iovannone and colleagues (2003) identified six core components that are critical to establishing comprehensive instructional programs for school-age children with ASD and their families. Table 12.5 summarizes the six key elements most likely to lead to a successful school-age educational experience for a child with ASD (Iovannone, Dunlap, Huber, & Kincaid, 2003).

The National Autism Center provides one of the most comprehensive reviews of evidence-based interventions (see www.nationalautismcenter.com) for children, adolescents, and young adults with ASD under the age of 22. In the most recent iteration of their National Standards Project (2015), a national panel identified 14 established interventions with sufficient evidence for effectiveness. Eighteen emerging interventions were identified with some evidence, but the evidence was considered insufficient. There were also 13 interventions considered unestablished as there was no current scientific evidence for their effectiveness. Many of these interventions are used by SLPs and other team members to support children with ASD. Table 12.6 outlines five interventions in the established category that would be most likely implemented by SLPs to support the language and

Table 12.5 Description of the core program components necessary for a positive school-age experience for children with ASD

Core components	Description
Individualized supports and services	Matches practices, services, and supports to a child's unique communication or learning profile, often through the IPE process Considers child and family preferences, strengths, and challenge areas requiring support
Systematic instruction	Requires planning, identifying valid goals, defining instructional procedures, evaluating effectiveness, and adjusting instruction as needed
Structured learning environment	Ensures curriculum is clear to both the children in the classroom and the staff supporting them (e.g., schedule of activities, choices, etc.)
Specialized curriculum content	Emphasizes social engagement, initiation and responding to social bids, as well as appropriate recreational and leisure skills
Functional approach to problem behavior	Focuses on replacing problem behavior with appropriate behavior
Family involvement	Includes collaboration with parents to ensure consistent instruction across settings

Adapted from Iovannone, Dunlap, Huber, and Kincaid (2003)

Table 12.6 Selected established interventions used by SLPs to support social communication and social interaction in children with ASD

Selected established interventions	Skills increased	Behaviors decreased	Ages
Naturalistic teaching strategies (e.g., focused stimulation, incidental and milieu teaching)	Communication, interpersonal, play Learning readiness	N/A	0–9
Joint attention intervention (e.g., response to social bids or initiation of bids)	Communication, interpersonal	N/A	0–5
Pivotal response training (e.g., pivotal targets, motivation, initiation, responsivity to multiple cues)	Communication, interpersonal, play Learning readiness	N/A	3–9
Language training (production) (e.g., modeling, prompting, cuing, reinforcing)	Communication, interpersonal, play	N/A	3–9
Parent training (e.g., expectant waiting, group training, joint attention, commenting, playdates)	Interpersonal, play	General symptoms Problem behaviors Restricted, repetitive, nonfunctional behavior, interests, or activity	0–18

social communication of children with ASD. It presents the skills typically increased and the behaviors that decrease when the intervention is implemented for children with ASD at particular ages.

There are a number of considerations families weigh when they are participating in intervention decision-making around their child with ASD. It is important that healthcare providers understand the perspectives that guide a family's willingness to move forward on an intervention approach. First, parents often choose interventions with and without an evidence base as their primary goal is always to ensure they are doing everything possible to help their child (Miller, Schreck, Mulick, & Butter, 2012). Second, most parents are not only concerned about the effectiveness of a treatment for their child but also the relationship they establish with the provider, whether or not they have access to the needed interventions, what the costs are, how medication fits into the care plan, and the family's general stress compounded by their child's limitations in communication, social interaction, and behavior (Mackintosh, Goin-Kochel, & Myers, 2012). The literature does tell us that the socioeconomic status of families influences their access to services (Irvin, McBee, Boyd, Hume, & Odom, 2012). In addition, families' treatment choices are affected by the severity of their child's sensory issues as parents will pursue intervention earlier, and those parents with a higher educational level often choose diet or vitamin treatments and access a greater number of services (Patten, Baranek, Watson, & Schultz, 2013). Ultimately, parents will generally pursue whatever is necessary for their child including complementary alternative approaches when traditional treatment shows limited progress (Herbert, 2014).

Summary

Although the incidence of ASD appears to have stabilized in the last 4 years, there has been a significant increase noted in the last 20 years, indicating the likelihood of multiple variables contributing to the condition. As a clinical diagnosis with a neurobiological basis, there are genetic and environmental influences that are likely to impact the expression of symptoms. Providers have a responsibility to screen for early markers of ASD and make appropriate referrals. Speech-language pathologists can be important partners in the screening, evaluation, and assessment process. Since communication disorders and intellectual disabilities can co-occur with ASD, and other conditions may share some of the symptoms of ASD, it is important that an experienced evaluation team is involved in the diagnosis of a child suspected autism. Early intervention is critical if a child is to achieve their full potential and providers have a responsibility for understanding the range of interventions and the available evidence for those interventions. Speech-language pathologists have a specific role in supporting the social communication and social interaction of children with ASD and are a crucial part of their educational team. Providers should also be aware that families consider a number of variables when making intervention decisions. It is important they are fully informed of their options and supported in the decisions they make.

References

Adamson, L. B., Deckner, D. F., & Bakeman, R. (2010). Early interests and joint engagement in typical development, autism & Down syndrome. *Journal of Autism & Developmental Disorders, 40*, 665–676.

Allison, C., Auyeung, B., & Baron-Cohen, S. (2012). Toward brief 'red flags' for autism screening: The short autism spectrum quotient and the short quantitative checklist in 1000 cases and 3000 controls. *Journal of the American Academy of Child & Adolescent Psychiatry, 51*(2), 202–212.

Allison, C., Baron-Cohen, S., Wheelwright, S., Charman, T., Richler, J., Pasco, G., & Brayne, C. (2008). A normally distributed quantitative measure of autism traits at 18-24 months of age: Preliminary report. *Journal of Autism & Developmental Disorders, 38*, 1414–1425.

American Psychiatric Association. (2013). *Diagnostic and statistical manual of mental disorders, DSM-5* (5 th ed.). Washington, DC: Author.

Bailey, A., Luthert, P., Dean, A., Harding, B., & Janota, I. (1998). A clinicopathological study of autism. *Brain, 121*, 889–905.

Baird, G., Charman, T., Baron-Cohen, S., Cox, A., Swettenham, J., Wheelright, S., et al. (2000). A screening instrument for autism at 18 months of age: A six-year follow-up study. *Journal of American Academy of Child Adolescent Psychiatry, 39*, 694–702.

Bakeman, R., & Adamson, L. (1984). Coordinating attention to people and objects in mother-infant and peer-infant interaction. *Child Development, 55*, 1278–1289.

Bang, J., Burns, J., & Nadig, A. (2013). Brief report: Conveying subjective experience in conversation: production of mental state terms and personal narratives in individuals with high functioning autism. *Journal of Autism & Developmental Disorders, 43*(7), 1732–1740.

Baranek, G. T. (1999). Autism during infancy: A retrospective video analysis of sensory-motor and social behaviors at 9-12 months of age. *Journal of Autism & Developmental Disorders, 29*, 213–224.

Baron-Cohen, S. (1987). Autism and symbolic play. *British Journal of Developmental Psychology, 5*, 139–148.

Baron-Cohen, S., Allen, J., & Gillberg, C. (1992). Can autism be detected at 18 months? The needle, the haystack, and the CHAT. *British Journal of Psychiatry, 161*, 839–843.

Baron-Cohen, S., Cox, A., Baird, G., Swettenham, J., Nightingale, N., Morgan, K., et al. (1996). Psychological markers in the detection of autism in infancy in a large population. *British Journal of Psychiatry, 168*, 138–163.

Baron-Cohen, S., Leslie, A. M., & Frith, U. (1986). Mechanical, behavioural and intentional understanding of picture stories in autistic children. *British Journal of Developmental Psychology, 4*, 113–125.

Barton, M., & Volkmar, F. R. (1998). How commonly are known medical conditions associated with autism? *Journal of Autism & Developmental Disorders, 28*, 273–278.

Bono, M., Daley, T., & Sigman, M. (2004). Relations among joint attention, amount of intervention and language gains in autism. *Journal of Autism & Developmental Disorders, 34*, 495–505.

Bopp, K. D., Mirenda, P., & Zumbo, B. D. (2009). Behavior predictors of language development over 2 years in children with ASD. *Journal of Speech, Language, Hearing Research, 52*, 1106–1120.

Capps, L., Yirmiya, N., & Sigman, M. (1992). Understanding of simple and complex emotions in non-retarded children with autism. *Journal of Child Psychology and Psychiatry, 33*, 1169–1182.

Centers for Disease Control (CDC). (2012). Autism and developmental disabilities monitoring network surveillance year 2008 principal investigators. Prevalence of autism spectrum disorders – autism and developmental disabilities monitoring network, 14 sites, United States, 2008. *Morbidity and Mortality 1655 Weekly Report, 61*(SS03), 1–19.

Centers for Disease Control (CDC). (2014). Autism and developmental disabilities monitoring network surveillance year 2010 principal investigators. prevalence of autism spectrum disorders among children aged 8 years—autism and developmental disabilities monitoring network, 11 sites, United States, 2010. *Morbidity and Mortality Weekly Report, 63*(2), 1–21.

Christensen, D. L., Baio, J., Van Naarden Braun, K., Bilder, D., Charles, J., Constantino, J. N., et al. (2016). Prevalence and Characteristics of Autism Spectrum Disorder Among Children Aged 8 Years — Autism and Developmental Disabilities Monitoring Network, 11 Sites, United States, 2012. *Surveillance Summaries, 65*(3), 1–23.

Christensen, D. L., Bilder, D. A., Zahorodny, W., Pettygrove, S., Durkin, M. S., Fitzgerald, R. T., et al. (2015). Prevalence and characteristics of ASD among 4-year-old children in the autism and developmental disabilities monitoring network. *Journal of Developmental & Behavioral Pediatrics 37*(1), 1–8.

Clifford, S., Young, R., & Williamson, P. (2007). Assessing the early characteristics of autistic disorder using video analysis. *Journal of Autism & Developmental Disorders, 37*, 301–313.

Clifford, S. M., & Dissanayake, C. (2008). The early development of joint attention to infants with autistic disorder using home video observation and parental interview. *Journal of Autism & Developmental Disorder, 38*, 791–805.

Coe, B. P., Girirajan, S., & Eichler, E. E. (2012). The genetic variability and commonality of neurodevelopmental disease. *American Journal of Medical Genetics Part C: Seminars in Medical 1418 Genetics, 160*(2), 118–129.

Colombi, C., Liebal, K., Tomasello, M., Young, G., Warneken, F., & Rogers, S. J. (2009). Examining correlates of cooperation in autism. Imitation, joint attention, and understanding intentions. *Autism, 13*(2), 143–163.

Constantino, J. N., Przybeck, T., Friesen, D., & Todd, R. D. (2000). Reciprocal social behavior in children with and without pervasive development disorders. *Developmental and Behavioral Pediatrics, 21*(1), 2–11.

Dawson, G., Toth, K., Abbott, R., Osterling, J., Munson, J., Estes, A., & Liaw, J. (2004). Early social attention impairments in autism: Social orienting, joint attention, and attention to distress. *Developmental Psychology, 40*(2), 271–283.

Dietz, C., Swinkels, S., van Daalen, E., van Engeland, H., & Buitelaar, J. K. (2006). Screening for autistic spectrum disorder in children aged 14-15 months II: Population screening with the *Early Screening of Autistic Traits Questionnaire* (ESAT). Design & general findings. *Journal of Autism & Developmental Disorders, 36*, 713–722.

Edelson, S. (2015). Genetics, the Environment, and Autism. e Autism Research Review International, 29 (3). Retrieved from http://www.autism.com/editorial_genes_edelson on January 9, 2016

Feldman, M. A., Ward, R. A., Savona, D., Regehr, K., Parker, K., Hudson, M., et al. (2012). Development and initial validation of a parent report measure of the behavioral development of infants at risk for autism spectrum disorders. *Journal of Autism & Developmental Disorders, 42*, 13–22.

Fernell, E., Hedvall, A., Norrelgen, F., Eriksson, M., Hoglund-Clarkson, L., Barnevik-Plsson, M., et al. (2010). Developmental profiles in preschool children with ASD referred for intervention. *Research in Developmental Disabilities, 31*, 790–799.

Geschwind, D. H. (2011). Genetics of autism spectrum disorders. *Trends in Cognitive Sciences, 15*(9), 409–416.

Giarelli, E., Wiggins, L. D., Rice, C. E., Levy, S. E., Kirby, R. S., Pinto-Martin, J., & Mandell, D. (2010). Sex differences in eth evaluation and diagnosis of autism spectrum disorders among children. *Disability & Health Journal, 3*, 107–116.

Hauck, M., Fein, D., Waterhouse, L., & Feinstein, C. (1995). Social initiations by autistic children to adults and other children. *Journal of Autism & Developmental Disorders, 25*(6), 579–595.

Hebert, E. B. (2014). Factors affecting parental decision-making regarding interventions for their child with autism. *Focus on Autism & Other Developmental Disabilities, 9*(2), 111–124.

Hobson, R. P., & Lee, A. (1998). Hello and goodbye: A study of social engagement in autism. *Journal of Autism and Developmental Disorders, 28*(2), 117–127.

Iovannone, R., Dunlap, G., Huber, H., & Kincaid, D. (2003). Effective educational practices for students with autism spectrum disorders. *Focus on Autism and Other Developmental Disabilities, 18*(3), 150–165.

Irvin, D. W., McBee, M., Boyd, B. A., Hume, K., & Odom, S. L. (2012). Child and family factors associated with the use of services for preschoolers with autism spectrum disorder. *Research in Autism Spectrum Disorders, 6*, 565–572.

Jarrold, C., Boucher, J., & Smith, P. (1993). Symbolic play in autism: A review. *Journal of Autism & Developmental Disorders, 23*(2), 281–307.

Johnson, C. P. (2008). Recognition of autism before age 2 years. *Pediatrics in Review, 29*, 86–96.

Johnson, C. P., Myers, S. M., & Council on Children with Disabilities. (2007). Identification and evaluation of children with autism spectrum disorders. *Pediatrics, 120*(5), 1183–1193.

Kasari, C., Chamberlain, B., & Bauminger, N. (2001). Social emotions and social relationships: Can children with autism compensate? In J. A. Burack, T. Charman, N. Yirmiya, & P. R. Zelazo (Eds.), *The development of autism: Perspective from theory and research* (pp. 309–323). Mahwah, NJ: Lawrence Erlbaum Associates.

Kasari, C., Sigman, M. D., Baumgartner, P., & Stipek, D. J. (1993). Pride and mastery in children with autism. *Journal of Child Psychology and Psychiatry, 34*, 353–362.

Kim, S. H., Paul, R., Tager-Flusberg, H., & Lord, C. (2014). Language and communication in autism. In F. R. Volkmar, S. J. Rogers, R. Paul, & K. A. Pelphrey (Eds.), *Handbook of autism and pervasive developmental disorders-4th edition, Volume 1: Diagnosis, development and brain mechanisms* (pp. 230–262). Hoboken, NJ: John Wiley & Sons.

Kim, S. H., Thurm, A., Shumway, S., & Lord, C. (2013). Multisite study of new *Autism Diagnostic Interview-Revised* (ADI-R) algorithms for toddlers and young preschoolers. *Journal of Autism & Developmental Disorders, 43*, 1527–1538.

Kleinman, J. M., Robins, D. L., Ventola, P. E., Pandey, J., Boorstein, H. C., Esser, E. L., et al. (2008). The *Modified Checklist for Autism in Toddlers*: A follow-up study investigating the early detection of ASD. *Journal of Autism & Developmental Disorders, 38*(5), 815–826.

Kozlowski, A. M., Matson, J. L., Worley, J. A., Sipes, M., & Horovitz, M. (2012). Defining characteristics for young children meeting cut off on the modified checklist for autism in toddlers. *Research in Autism Spectrum Disorders, 6*, 472–479.

Lewis, V., & Boucher, J. (1988). Spontaneous, instructed and elicited play in relatively able autistic children. *British Journal of Developmental Psychology, 6*, 325–339.

Lord, C. (1995). Follow-up of two-year-olds referred for possible autism. *J. Child Psychol Psychiatry, 36*, 1365–1382.

Lord, C., Luyster, R.J., Gotham K., & Guthrie, W. (2013). *Autism Diagnostic Observation Schedule (ADOS-2)-Toddler Module.* Los Angeles, CA: Western Psychological Services.

Lord, C., & Magill, J. (1989). Methodological and theoretical issues in studying peer-directed behavior in autism. In G. Dawson (Ed.), *Autism: Nature, diagnosis and treatment* (pp. 326–345). New York: Guilford Press.

Lord, C., Rutter, M., DiLavore, P. C., Risi, S., Gotham, K., & Bishop, S. L. (2013). *Autism Diagnostic Observation Schedule (ADOS-2)*, 2nd ed. Los Angeles, CA: Western Psychological Services.

Lord, C., Rutter, M., & LeCouteur, A. (1994). Autism Diagnostic Interview-Revised: A revised version of a diagnostic interview for caregivers of individuals with possible pervasive developmental disorders. *Journal of Autism & Developmental Disorders, 24*(5), 659–685.

Loveland, K. A., & Landry, S. H. (1986). Joint attention and language in autism and developmental language delay. *Journal of Autism & Developmental Disorders, 16*, 335–349.

Mackintosh, V. A., Goin-Kochel, R. P., & Myers, B. J. (2012). "What do you like/dislike about the treatments you're currently using?": A qualitative study of parents of children with autism spectrum disorders. *Focus on Autism & Other Developmental Disabilities, 27*(1), 51–60.

Mars, A. E., Mauk, J. E., & Dowrick, P. W. (1998). Symptoms of pervasive developmental disorders as observed in prediagnostic home videos of infants and toddlers. *Journal of Pediatrics, 132*, 500–504.

Matson, J. L., Wilkins, J., & Fodstad, J. C. (2011). The validity of the baby and toddler screen for children with autism traits: Part 1 (BISCUIT: Part 1). *Journal of Autism & Developmental Disorders, 41*(9), 1139–1146.

Mildenberger, K., Sitter, S., Noterdaeme, M., & Amorosa, H. (2001). The use of the ADI-R as a diagnostic tool in the differential diagnosis of children with infantile autism and children with a receptive language disorder. *European Child & Adolescent Psychiatry, 10*, 248–255.

Miller, V. A., Schreck, K. A., Mulick, J. A., & Butter, E. (2012). Factors related to parents' choices of treatments for their children with autism spectrum disorders. *Research in Autism Spectrum Disorders, 6*, 87–95.

Mundy, P., & Sigman, M. (1989). Specifying the nature of the social impairment in autism. In G. Dawson (Ed.), *Autism: Nature, diagnosis and treatment* (pp. 3–21). New York: Guilford Press.

Mundy, P., Sigman, M., & Kasari, C. (1990). A longitudinal study of joint attention and language development in autistic children. *Journal of Autism & Developmental Disorders, 20*, 115–128.

Murray, D. S., Creaghead, N. A., Maning-Courtney, P., Shear, P. K., Bean, J., & Prendeville, J. (2008). The relationship between joint attention and language in children with autism spectrum disorders. *Focus on Autism & Other Developmental Disabilities, 23*(1), 5–14.

National Autism Center (2015). *National Standards Project, Phase 2: Addressing the need for evidence-based practice guidelines for ASD.* (www.nationalautismcenter.org)

National Research Council. (2001). *Educating children with autism. Committee on Educational Interventions for Children with Autism: Division of Behavioral and Social Sciences and Education*. Washington, DC: National Academy Press.

Neale, B. M., Kou, Y., Liu, L., Ma'ayan, A., Samocha, K. E., Sabo, A., et al. (2012). Patterns and rates of exonic de novo mutations in autism spectrum disorders. *Nature, 485*(7397), 242–245.

O'Roak, B. J., Vives, L., Fu, W., Egertson, J. D., Stanaway, I. B., Phelps, I. G., et al. (2012). Multiplex targeted sequencing identifies recurrently mutated genes in autism spectrum disorders. 1578. *Science, 338*(6114), 1619–1622.

Osterling, J., & Dawson, G. (1994). Early recognition of children with autism: A study of first birthday home videotapes. *Journal of Autism & Developmental Disorders, 24, 247–258.*

Ozonoff, S., Losif, A.-M., Baguio, F., Cook, I. C., Hill, M. M., Hutman, T., et al. (2010). A prospective study of the emergence of early behavioral signs of autism. *Journal of the American Academy of Child & Adolescent Psychiatry, 49*(3), 256–266.

Patten, E., Baranek, G. T., Watson, L. B., & Schultz, B. (2013). Child and family characteristics influencing intervention choices in autism spectrum disorders. *Focus on Autism & Othere Developmental Disabilities, 28*(3), 138–146.

Paul, R., & Fahim, D. (2014). Assessing communication in ASD. In F. R. Volkmar, S. J. Rogers, R. Paul, & K. A. Pelphrey (Eds.), *Handbook of autism and pervasive developmental disorders-4th edition, Volume 2: Assessment, interventions and policy* (pp. 673–694). Hoboken, NJ: John Wiley & Sons.

Rapin, I., & Tuchman, R. F. (2008). Autism: Definition, neurobiology, screening, diagnosis. *Pediatric Clinics in North America, 55*, 1129–1146.

Robins, D. L., Fein, D., Barton, M. L., & Green, J. A. (2001). The Modified Checklist for Autism in Toddlers: An initial study investigating the early detection of Autism and Pervasive Developmental Disorders. *Journal of Autism & Developmental Disorders, 31*(2), 131–144.

Rogers, S. J., Hepburn, S. L., Stackhouse, T., & Wehner, E. (2003). Imitation performance in toddlers with autism and those with other developmental disorders. *Journal of Child Psychology and Psychiatry, 44*(5), 763–781.

Sanders, S. J., Murtha, M. T., Gupta, A. R., Murdoch, J. D., Raubeson, M. J., Willsey, A. J., et al. (2012). De novo mutations revealed by whole-exome sequencing are strongly associated with autism. 1628. *Nature, 485*(7397), 237–241.

Scarpa, A., Reyes, N. M., Patriquin, M. A., Lorenzi, J., Hasssenfeldt, T. A., Desai, V. J., & Kerkering, K. W. (2013). The Modified Checklist for Autism in Toddler: Reliability in a diverse rural American sample. *Journal of Autism & Developmental Disorders, 43*, 2269–2279.

Shumway, S., & Wetherby, A. M. (2009). Communicative acts of children with ASD in the second year of life. *Journal of Speech, Language, Hearing Research, 52*, 1139–1156.

Shumway, S., Wetherby, A.M., & Woods, J. (2003, November). *Red flags of autism spectrum disorders in the second and third years of life.* Paper presented at the Annual Convention of the American Speech-Language-Hearing Association, Chicago, IL.

Sigman, M., & Ungerer, J. (1984). Attachment behaviors in autistic children. *Journal of Autism and Developmental Disorders, 14*, 231–244.

Sigman, M., Ungerer, J., Mundy, P., & Sherman, T. (1987). Cognition in autistic children. In D. Cohen, A. Donnellan, & R. Paul (Eds.), *Handbook of autism and atypical developmental disorders* (pp. 103–120). New York: John Wiley & Sons.

Smith, I. C., Reichow, B., & Volkmar, F. (2015). The effects of DSM-5 criteria on number of individuals diagnosed with ASD: A systematic review. *Journal of Autism & Developmental Disorders, 45*, 2541–2552.

St. Georges, C., Cassel, R.S., Cohen, D., Chetouani, M., Lasnik, M.C., Maestro, S., & Muratori, F. (2010). What studies of family home movies can teach us about autistic infants. *Research in Autism Spectrum Disorders, 4*, 355–366.

Szymanski, C.A., Brice, P.J., Lam, K.H., & Hotto, S. A. (2012). Deaf children with autism spectrum disorders. *Journal of Autism and Developmental Disorders, 42*(10), 2027–2037.

Tager-Flusberg, H., Rogers, S., Cooper, J., Landa, R., Lord, C., Paul, R., et al. (2009). Defining spoken language benchmarks and selecting measures of expressive language development for young children with ASD. *Journal of Speech, Language, Hearing Research, 52*, 643–652.

Tomasello, M. (1995). Joint attention as social cognition. In C. Moore & P. J. Dunham (Eds.), *Joint attention, its origins and role in development*. Hillsdale, NJ: Lawrence Erlbaum.

Trillingsgaard, A., Sorensen, E. U., Nemec, G., & Jorgensen, M. (2005). What distinguishes autism spectrum disorders from other developmental disorders before the age of four years? *European Journal of Child and Adolescent Psychiatry, 14*, 65–72.

Uljarevic, M., & Hamilton, A. (2013). Recognition of emotions in autism: A formal meta-analysis. *Journal of Autism and Developmental Disorders, 43*(7), 1517–1526.

Ventola, P., Kleinman, J., Pandey, P., Wilson, L., Esser, E., Boorstein, H., et al. (2007). Differentiating between autism spectrum disorders and other developmental disabilities in children who failed a screening instrument for ASD. *Journal of Autism and Developmental Disorders, 37*, 4325–4436.

Werner, E., Dawson, G., Osterling, J., & Dinno, N. (2000). Brief report: Recognition of autism spectrum disorder before one year of age: A retrospective study based on home videotapes. *Journal of Autism and Developmental Disorders, 30*, 157–158.

Wetherby, A. M., Watt, N., Morgan, L., & Shumway, S. (2007). Social communication profiles of children with autism spectrum disorders late in the second year of life. *Journal of Autism & Development Disorders, 37*, 960–975.

Wetherby, A. M., & Woods, J. (2002). *Systematic Observation of Red Flags for Autism Spectrum Disorders in Young Children (SORF), Unpublished manual*. Tallahassee, FL: Florida State University.

Wetherby, A. M., & Woods, J. (2003, November). *Red flags of autism spectrum disorders in the second year of life*. Paper presented at the Annual Convention of the American Speech-Language-Hearing Association, Chicago, IL.

Wetherby, A. M., Woods, J., Allen, L., Cleary, J., Dickinson, H., & Lord, C. (2004). Early indicators of ASD in the second year of life. *Journal of Autism & Developmental Disorders 34*(5), 1–22.

Yirmiya, N., Sigman, M., Kasari, C., & Mundy, P. (1992). Empathy and cognition in high-functioning children with autism. *Child Development, 63*, 150–160.

Young, R. L., & Rodi, M. L. (2014). Redefining ASD using DSM-5: The implications of the proposed DSM-5 criteria for ASD. *Journal of Autism & Developmental Disorders, 44*, 758–765.

Index

P. A. Prelock, T. L. Hutchins, *Clinical Guide to Assessment and Treatment of Communication Disorders*, Best Practices in Child and Adolescent Behavioral Health Care, https://doi.org/10.1007/978-3-319-93203-3

B

C

T

The manufacturer's authorised representative in the EU is Springer Nature Customer Service Centre GmbH, Europaplatz 3, 69115 Heidelberg, Germany. If you have any concerns regarding our products, please contact ProductSafety@springernature.com

Printed and bound by CPI Group (UK) Ltd, Croydon, CR0 4YY
30/09/2026
02225258-0010